1 6 JUN 2007

28 JUL 2007

- 1 APR 2008

- 8 ⁱ - 2009

15. MAR 10.

- 5 MAY 2011

1 0 NOV 2011

1 9 SEP 2012

- 6 MAR 2013

03 JUN 2014

3 1 AUG 2015

1 4 SEP 2015

1 6 JAN 2016

18.02.14

~~1 MAR 2017~~

- 1 MAR 2017

2 7 SEP 2018

2 8 MAR 2019

1 4 DEC 2019

SANTON, Kate

Calorie
counting

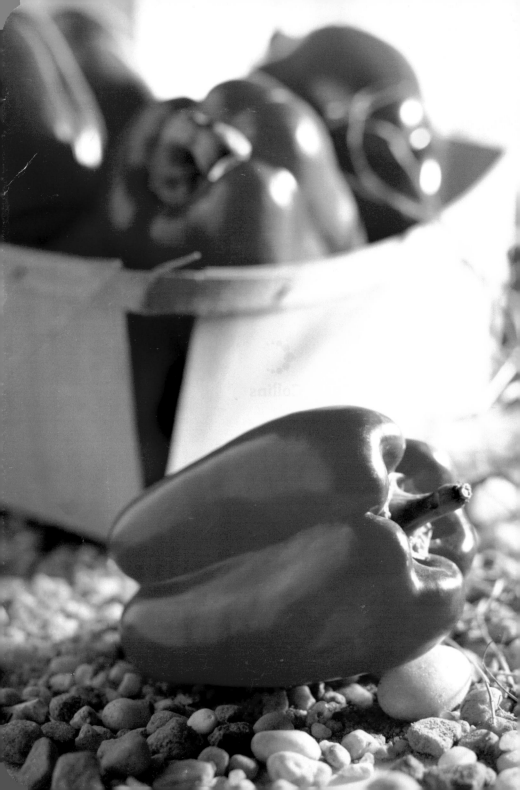

need to know?

Calorie
Counting

Collins

First published in 2007 by Collins
an imprint of
HarperCollins Publishers
77–85 Fulham Palace Road
London W6 8JB

www.collins.co.uk

A catalogue record for this book is available from
the British Library

Text: Kate Santon
Editor: Grapevine Publishing Services
Designer: Judith Ash
Series design: Mark Thomson
Front cover photograph: Alamy
Back cover photographs: Jupiter Images (all three)

ISBN-13: 978-0-00-724664-9
ISBN-10: 0-00-724664-1

Colour reproduction by Colourscan, Singapore
Printed and bound by Printing Express Ltd,
Hong Kong

Contents

Introduction 7

1   **How does calorie counting work?** 9

2   **Assessing the situation** 23

3   **Improving energy out** 39

4   **Improving energy in** 59

5   **Calorie counting in practice** 87

6   **Menu suggestions** 115

7   **Recipes** 125

8   **Listings** 157

Appendices 187

Further reading 188

Useful addresses 189

Picture credits 190

Index 191

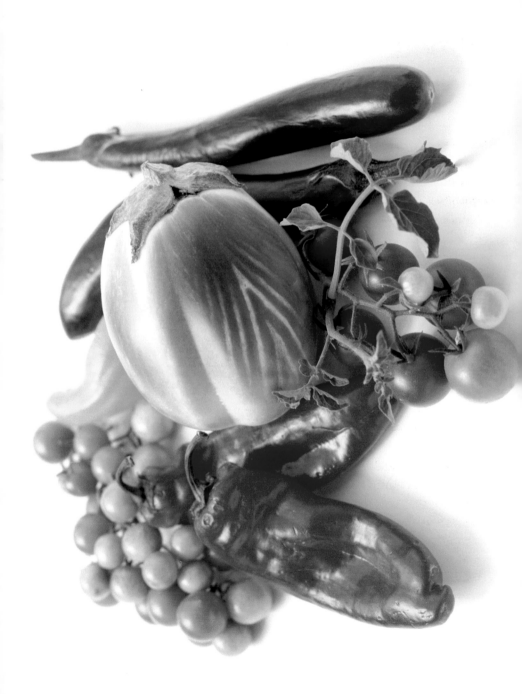

Introduction

Sometimes it seems as though every day brings another diet.
They are all supposed to be effective, and they are all supposed
to be easy. The fact is, however, that many are neither. When it
comes down to it, there's only one sure way to lose weight and
keep it off: eat less and do more. It's all down to calories.

Calories are a simple measure of energy; like all living things,
and like machines, we need energy to function. Breathing,
moving about, digesting food – bodily processes are all
dependent on energy, and that energy comes from the food and
drink we consume. Most diets restrict calories in some shape or
form, whether they are sensible, balanced diets or fad diets that
focus on one type of food. They might do it by substituting some
meals with special foods or by restricting the types of food
eaten, but the general aim is to reduce the calories taken in.

The advantage of calorie counting over other diets is the
freedom – and the flexibility – it brings. It is freedom with some
structure or it wouldn't work, but no one is going to tell you
exactly what to eat and when; you work that out for yourself.
You can be creative, and adapt your diet to suit your lifestyle,
while eating healthily and keeping tally.

Controlling your weight is perfectly possible, and you don't
need to feel deprived, bored or make yourself ill. You can re-train
your body in the process. Of course, counting calories does call
for a conscious effort but – and this is the biggest advantage –
it can really help you to lose weight and keep it off long term.

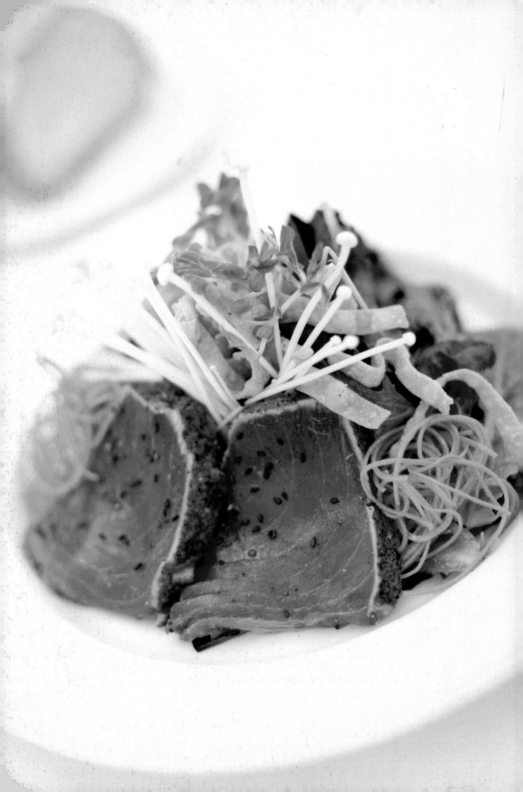

1 How does calorie counting work?

If you want to lose weight then you need to take in less energy than you use, and that means fewer calories in the form of food and drink. When you take in less energy than your body needs, stored energy has to be used instead – generally energy stored in the form of body fat – a process known as 'burning fat'. Time for a little bit of useful science.

How does calorie counting work?

Getting your energy in/energy out balance right is the key to understanding weight loss, and making counting calories work for you. This chapter explains how.

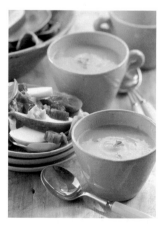

Home-made soup is ideal for a calorie-controlled lunch.

What is a calorie?

One calorie is a measure that represents a tiny amount of energy, so 'kilocalories' are generally used instead by scientists and nutritionists. A single kilocalorie (kCal), or a thousand calories, is the amount of energy required to raise the temperature of a fixed quantity of water by $1°C$, from $14.5°C$ to $15.5°C$. The term kilocalorie is more often seen on packaging than it is used in everyday life, and the word 'calorie' has come to be widely used to mean the same thing, which is how it is used in this book. Sometimes the two are written with a capital letter.

You might also see 'kJ' on packaging, which stands for 'kilojoule', another measurement of energy. One kilocalorie equals approximately 4.18 kilojoules, and the term kilojoule is beginning to replace kilocalorie in some places, so you may well see that appearing more often.

You might also have seen references to 'fat calories' and 'carbohydrate calories', and suggestions that some are worse than others. However, in practice – and under normal living conditions, not extreme survival situations – there's no real difference. So a thousand calories from butter, a thousand from bread, a thousand from beef and a thousand from broad beans will have similar effects on your overall weight, though they may not have similar effects on your health, of course. The way calories are made available to your body – the food choices you make – can make a difference, however; a meal that leaves you feeling satisfied and which fends off the return of hunger is ideal as it doesn't tempt you into eating again quickly, or eating more than you need in the first place.

How to use your body's responses: energy in

Most food is digested in the small intestine apart from 'simple' sugars and alcohol, which are digested in the stomach itself. During the process of digestion, all food is broken down so that the body can use it. A lot of what we eat is converted into glucose, one of those 'simple' sugars that is

must know

Weight fluctuations

Perfectly normal fluctuations in your weight can be discouraging, so don't get on the scales every day. Weigh yourself regularly if you wish, but not more than once a week. Once a fortnight is fine.

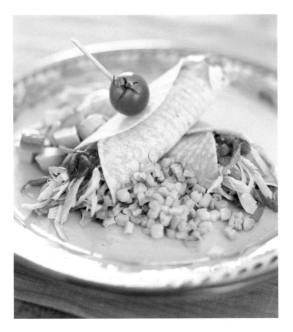

Serving lighter meals with extra vegetables helps balance your diet – and fill you up.

must know

Stress eating

If you are stressed,
depressed or bored,
then crisps or chocolate
aren't going to solve the
underlying problem.
In fact, they'll probably
make you more stressed
and depressed because
you've weakened your
resolve; try to address
what's really wrong.

absorbed very quickly and easily. Some of the glucose that enters the bloodstream is used immediately, some is stored in the liver and muscles as glycogen, and any surplus is converted into fat – and stored.

Because glucose is digested in the stomach it enters the bloodstream quickly and the quantity of glucose in the blood soars. This results in a rapid rise in blood-sugar levels, sometimes called a 'spike'. One of the problems associated with this is that it is followed by an equally swift drop, which prompts your body to boost glucose levels again, making you feel hungrier than before. The rise in blood sugar also generates a matching rise in insulin, a hormone produced by the pancreas that enables glucose to enter the body's cells.

In recent years, with the rise in popularity of GI/GL diets, we have come to realize that it's not just diabetics (who lack insulin) who need to keep blood-sugar levels steady. It is critical for your health, not just for weight loss. More and more people are developing insulin resistance syndrome, and one of the major risk factors for this is being overweight. In insulin resistance syndrome the body fails to respond to insulin properly so the pancreas produces more and more to compensate. This is not good: it has been linked to high blood pressure, type 2 diabetes (also called adult-onset diabetes), heart disease and even some cancers, so it is really worth trying to prevent it from developing in the first place.

There's yet another reason to keep insulin levels steady: if they are fluctuating, it can inhibit the release of stored fat, which is just what you don't want when you are trying to control your weight.

Stabilizing insulin levels means stabilizing blood-sugar levels, and stabilizing blood-sugar levels means, as far as your day-to-day weight-loss efforts go, that you'll feel less hungry. The trick is to eat fewer of the foods that cause blood-sugar spikes and learn how to moderate the effects. Doing this can be comparatively simple; it could mean, for example, consuming more fibre by eating a whole apple rather than a peeled one.

There's one other point to bear in mind about blood sugar and insulin. The more muscle cells you have, particularly toned muscle, the more effectively you use glucose and insulin. Fat cells don't use them efficiently. So the greater your ratio of muscle to fat, the better. It all works together.

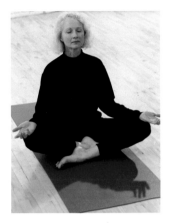

Meditation reduces blood pressure, heart rate and breathing rate and is a good method of controlling stress.

How to use your body's responses: energy out

The other side of the energy balance is a little more complicated, and not so obvious. Our bodies 'burn off' energy in three basic ways.

RMR

The most important way in which energy is burned in the body involves the resting metabolic rate or RMR. This accounts for about 65–75 per cent of the total energy used by the body; in fact some sources put it as high as 80 per cent. This is also sometimes called the basal metabolic rate, but whatever it's called it means the same thing: the energy used by your body even when you are totally at rest, the minimum energy it needs just to tick over. These calories are used to fuel processes like the circulation of the blood, breathing, sending messages to

must know

Slip-ups

Forgive yourself if you drift off your diet. Everyone does at some time, but feeling horrible about yourself doesn't help. Just make sure it doesn't become a habit or you'll undermine your dieting confidence.

and from the brain, keeping your body temperature stable – your body's basic functions. They are the involuntary processes that by definition don't require conscious control; the things you are, by and large, almost unaware of your body doing.

Everyone's RMR is different. There's a genetic element, but there are other variables. In some circumstances, for instance, the body's involuntary processes require more energy. Your RMR increases during periods of rapid growth. The need for more energy while pregnant or breastfeeding is fairly obvious, but the need for extra energy if you are recovering from surgery or an injury of some kind is perhaps less so. In those cases more calories are needed for the body's repair mechanisms to function. RMR decreases with age and is at its highest in children below the age of 10, who have a lot of growing to do.

It varies in other ways, too. Most significantly for dieters, muscle uses more energy than fat. This is an important factor because a kilogram of muscle can burn more than 120 kCal a day at rest, whereas a kilogram of fat would only require about 20. So if you are fit, your body will use more energy even when you are just sitting still than it would if you were unfit. Muscle requires more energy than fat to keep going. The more muscle you have, the better the overall effect on your RMR. That's the reason why men have a higher RMR than women: they usually have greater muscle mass. It's also one of the reasons why RMR declines with age, as older people have a tendency to lose muscle mass as well as slow down generally. This gradual drop in RMR begins relatively early in life: it's been suggested that it declines by 2 per cent for each decade after the age of 20.

The RMR is one of the reasons why crash diets are a bad idea: your body can't differentiate between a deliberate, very low-calorie diet and accidental or induced starvation, so it slows down your metabolism and hangs onto its fat reserves tenaciously to ensure its survival. If food is scarce, the body adapts to make the best use of what food it does get.

Exercise is an important part of any weight-loss programme and will help you to keep the weight off afterwards as well.

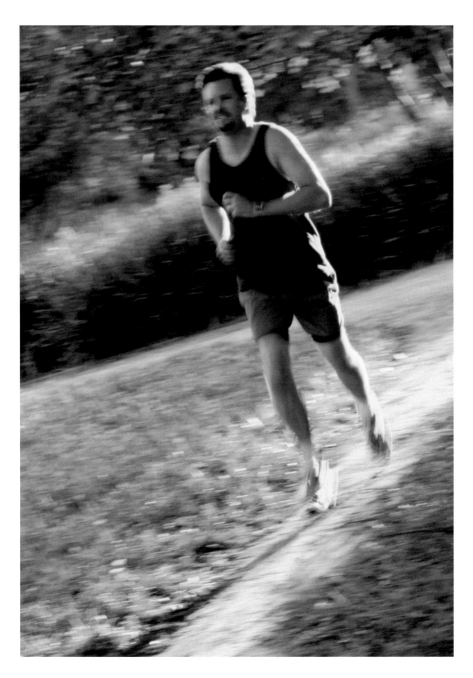

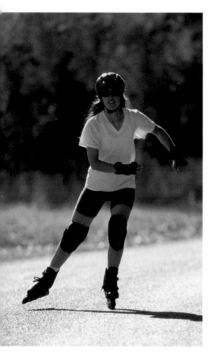

Rollerblading tones the waist, hip and leg muscles.

There's another RMR-related reason why weight loss should be gradual. Some of the weight you lose will come from lean muscle tissue, and if you lose weight speedily the proportion of lean-tissue loss is greater, and muscle uses more energy. As you lose weight, your RMR will drop to suit your new weight anyway – it takes more energy to keep a larger body going – but there's no reason to make that drop bigger than it need be. Remember that your RMR accounts for at least 65 to 75 per cent of the energy you use, and you will understand how important it is to prevent it from dropping unnecessarily.

Your RMR is also a reason why weight loss can slow down or stall, and it plays a part in explaining why it can be difficult to lose weight if you have dieted repeatedly in the past. When the RMR drops, you need fewer calories to keep going; any excess is simply deposited as fat and you put weight on. So the temptation is to diet again, and again the same thing happens – only this time you don't lose all the weight you gained because your RMR is slowing. It is often said that 'dieting makes you fat' because of the effects of this type of yo-yo dieting.

Finally, there are some metabolism myths you've probably come across. One of the most popular is that overweight people have a 'slow metabolism'. While it is true that metabolism varies from individual to individual, this is one sweeping generalization that isn't borne out by evidence. Most of the time a larger body requires more energy for basic functions: it's just got more work to do, so its RMR is actually greater. Metabolism will adjust to body size; if someone does manage to lose a lot of weight, then their metabolism adjusts downwards to a level appropriate for their new weight. It is possible, though, that an underactive thyroid, rather than a slow metabolism, might be playing a part if you are finding it very difficult to lose weight despite your best efforts. This only affects a small percentage of people, but it is worth asking your doctor to refer you for a blood test if you are concerned.

Some diets advertise that following their particular regime or eating their specific foods will increase your metabolic rate. Treat these claims with scepticism and remember that your RMR will inevitably fall as you lose weight. The only effective way of boosting your RMR is by becoming more active generally in everyday life and doing some regular structured exercise.

must know

Burn more fat

Boost your RMR by building muscle. Check out www.netfit.co.uk for some simple ideas and straightforward workouts.

The thermic effect of food

The second way in which your body uses energy is relatively simple. The thermic effect of food is the increase in energy above your RMR when you eat and digest food, and when your body stores the resulting energy. It varies but is generally around 10 per cent of the calorie value of the food eaten, so if you've just eaten a 500-calorie dinner, your body will use 50 calories to process it.

The thermic effect of exercise

The third way in which your body uses energy is in exercise. This doesn't just mean activities you might immediately think of when the word 'exercise' is mentioned – like cycling, weight training, running – but covers all activity over and above your RMR. If you walk to work, it counts; if you swim, it counts. If you are relatively sedentary, exercise could account for 10 per cent of your energy output, but if you are an athlete it could be up to 50 per cent - it's the most variable factor. How much energy you use doing any form of exercise is dependent on several factors, including your sex and weight, and may be surprisingly low: you'll find a chart showing the calories burned by some common activities in chapter 3, page 42.

In most circumstances (unless you're an international-level sportsperson) your RMR is by far and away the most significant part of your energy expenditure, so the best strategy for using more calories is to boost your RMR. Building more muscle mass while reducing your fat levels and developing a generally more active lifestyle - and making that a permanent part of your life, not just a temporary weight-loss tactic - is your best bet.

How much energy do you need?

Calculating your actual energy requirements can be problematic. There are many ways, ranging from complicated equations that allow for every variable, to basic generalizations giving one figure for men and another for women. When it comes down to it, they can all be very subjective: the word 'sedentary', for example, can be used to mean anything from having an office job to being bedridden, and putting the same basic figures through five different equations can give you five different answers.

Having said that, you *can* get a basic idea, a rough figure to use as a guideline. Try this:
• If you are a woman with a sedentary lifestyle (desk job, getting very limited exercise), multiply your weight in kilos by 26 to get an approximation of the

number of calories you are using per day. This is also the number of calories you would need to consume per day to maintain your current weight.

• If you are a similarly inactive man, multiply your weight in kilos by 31.

• If you are a moderately active woman (getting 60 minutes of moderate-intensity exercise a day – and remember the broad definition of exercise on page 17 – plus three weekly sessions of aerobic exercise like swimming, skipping or even dancing), multiply your weight in kilos by 33.

• If you are a moderately active man, multiply your weight in kilos by 37.

• If you're a very active woman (getting your daily 60 minutes of moderate-intensity exercise, and having 5–7 sessions of aerobic exercise every week), multiply your weight in kilos by 39.

• If you're a very active man, then multiply your weight in kilos by 44.

It has been calculated that a kilogram of weight is equivalent to about 7,000–7,700 calories. Many experts recommend that you don't try to lose more than 0.5kg a week, and to do this you'd need to take in approximately 3,500 calories fewer in a week than you do at present (i.e. about 500 calories a day).

However, if your calorie-expenditure calculations based on the formula above give a figure of less than 1500, dropping as much as 500 calories a day could push your overall calorie intake down too far. It is very important not to eat too little; that cannot be stressed enough. Very low calorie intake can induce a pattern of yo-yo dieting, as it's hard to stick with a diet that leaves you hungry. Your blood-sugar levels will be all over the place, leading to hunger, food

must know

Malnutrition

Watch out for signs that you are eating or drinking too little. Undue tiredness, weakness, headaches and confusion are extreme ones, but there are others. Check your nails, for instance. Brittle nails often indicate a lack of calcium, small white spots are a sign of zinc deficiency and fine white bands can mean you're not getting enough protein. Eating a balanced diet will correct all of these.

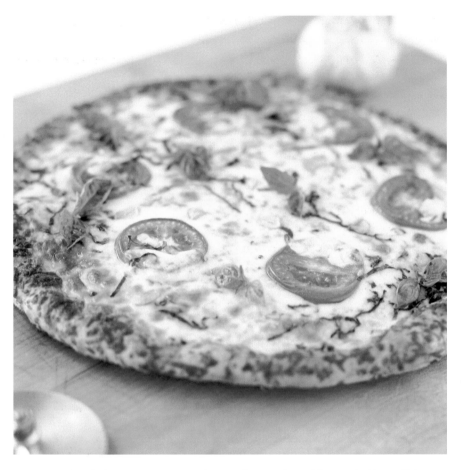

Pizza can blow your diet. Keep it for special occasions and go for the thin-crust ones without loads of toppings.

cravings and an unstoppable urge to binge. Going very low can also lead to malnutrition and all sorts of unwanted side effects (see the box on page 19).

On the other hand, this figure also illustrates how easy it is to put weight on. Eating 500 calories a day more than you need is worryingly simple; you might not even notice. Have garlic bread with cheese in a pizza restaurant, and you've eaten more than 500 calories in one go. But you don't do that every day, of course.

If you start your day with a Starbucks latte and a honey raisin bran muffin, that would come to over 600 calories. Add another latte at lunchtime, maybe one in the afternoon to keep you going... Being good and ordering chicken tikka instead of a rich curry in sauce is great, but avoid the naan if you don't want to undermine your good resolve – 160g of plain naan (one large piece) can be over 350 calories. A couple of large glasses of wine and a nibble at some nuts? Well, that's at least 500 calories, probably much more; the wine alone could be 340.

Fortunately it's not difficult to become calorie-aware, and there are lots of tips and suggestions in chapters 4 and 5.

Every individual is different, and it is hard to come up with a simple formula that is applicable to everyone, so many dietitians prefer to base their recommendations for appropriate weight-loss calorie intake on another factor: how much weight you have to lose.

want to know more?

• See chapter 2 for information on calculating how much you should aim to lose.
• If you are worried that you might have an underactive thyroid, see your doctor – a simple blood test will give you the answer.
• There's plenty of advice about healthy eating in chapter 4.

websites

• There is lots of sensible information online. A good place to start is www.bbc.co.uk/health/healthy_living.
• www.weightconcern.co.uk
• www.weightloss resources.co.uk
• www.sainsburys.com/healthyeating
• www.calorielab.com

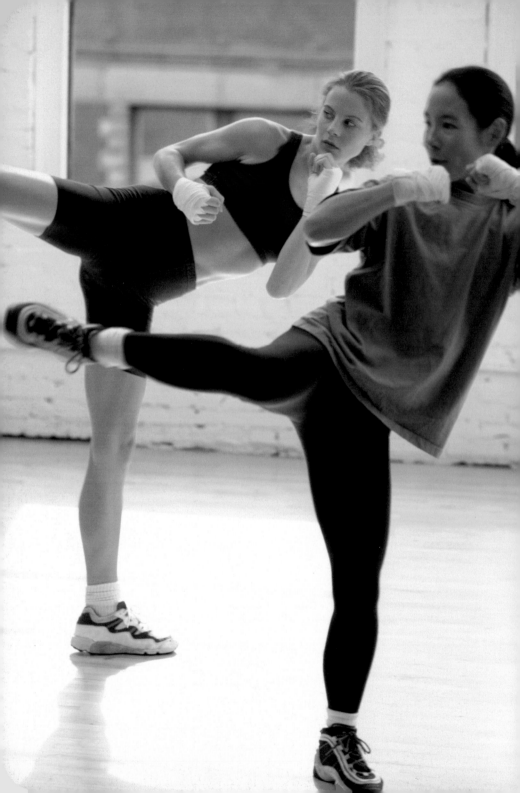

2 Assessing the situation

When you are contemplating dieting it is vital to have as realistic a picture as possible of what you are aiming for, and of what you can hope to achieve. Trying to get that picture by assessing your RMR is fraught with problems, as we've seen, though you can get a rough idea. In fact there's no definitive, utterly reliable method – but that doesn't mean there's nothing that can help.

Assessing the situation

Everyone has a natural weight range, a weight at which they feel most comfortable. If you diet down below yours, you'll find your new low weight almost impossible to maintain. Unfortunately it is much easier to maintain a weight above your natural range...

must know

Aim small

There's nothing wrong with aiming small – in fact it's best. Even minor losses in weight can result in better health, and losing little by little, over time, means you're more likely to keep the weight off permanently.

What sort of build are you?

When you are considering what weight to aim at, it's vital that you are sensible and realistic. One of the first steps is to take a clear look at how big you are. Not how heavy you are, but whether you have a naturally small, medium or large frame. If you fall into the latter category, you'll never succeed in turning yourself into someone with a small frame; it's not going to happen.

It's important not to make assumptions when assessing yourself, so work it out; many people assume that because they are tall or short they automatically have either a large or a small frame, and that's not the case.

To do this properly, you'll need to know your height in metres. Again, no assumptions: measure yourself against a door frame or wall, without shoes, and keep a note of your metric height. Once you know that, use a soft tape measure – not the stiff, DIY type – to measure around your wrist at the narrowest part. One of your wrists, depending on whether you are right- or left-handed, may well be slightly larger than the other; use the smaller one. Then check your height and wrist measurement against the chart opposite to find your frame size.

What is your frame size?

Women

Below 1.58m tall:
• Wrist measuring less than 14cm – small frame
• Wrist measuring between 14 and 15cm – medium frame
• Wrist measuring more than 15cm – large frame

1.58-1.65m tall:
• Wrist measuring less than 15cm – small frame
• Wrist measuring between 15 and 16cm – medium frame
• Wrist measuring more than 16cm – large frame

Above 1.65m tall:
• Wrist measuring less than 16cm – small frame
• Wrist measuring between 16 and 17cm – medium frame
• Wrist measuring more than 17cm – large frame

Men:

Below 1.65m tall:
• Wrist measuring less than 16cm – small frame
• Wrist measuring between 16 and 17cm – medium frame
• Wrist measuring more than 17cm – large frame

Above 1.65m tall:
• Wrist measuring less than 17cm – small frame
• Wrist measuring between 17 and 19cm – medium frame
• Wrist measuring more than 19cm – large frame

Now you know. Some of our proportions are simply genetic, and we'll never alter them. If you are just over 5ft tall – 1.54m – and have a large frame, you will never permanently transform yourself into a fragile little waif despite your height, and there's no point in trying to do so. If you do manage to lose a lot of weight you'll be unlikely to keep it off, and you probably won't look quite right either. So save yourself a lot of trouble by being realistic.

must know

Working out BMI

If you want a precise BMI figure, divide your weight in kilograms by the square of your height in metres, as in this example of someone 1.63m tall, who weighs 67kg:

$1.63 \times 1.63 = 2.65$
$67 \div 2.65 = 25.28$
The BMI is 25.28.

Height, weight, and the Body Mass Index

The next step is to consult a good height and weight chart, like the one opposite. This will give you some idea of what an 'ideal' weight for your height and frame would be, but it's just an approximation that mirrors a cultural average. Many factors can distort it, such as how athletic you are; muscle weighs more than fat, so some ballerinas would appear to be overweight using such charts. For those who aren't in that category of fitness, it can provide a guide.

You can add more information to help. Many GPs and dietitians are likely to use the body mass index to assess weight levels. It does have some of the same problems as a height and weight chart since it is culturally specific and doesn't consider the

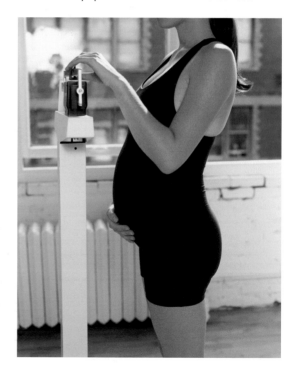

During pregnancy you should expect to put on about 11–16 kg if you had an 'average' BMI beforehand, 12–18 kg if you were underweight and 7–11 kg if you were overweight.

Standard body weight for height and frame size

Men

Height m (ft)	Small frame kg (lbs)	Medium frame kg (lbs)	Large frame kg (lbs)
1.60 (5'3")	51–61 (113–134)	54–64 (119–140)	58–68 (127–150)
1 63 (5'4")	53–61 (116–135)	55–65 (122–142)	59–70 (131–154)
1.65 (5'5")	54–62 (119–137)	57–66 (125–146)	60–72 (133–159)
1.68 (5'6")	56–64 (123–140)	59–68 (129–149)	62–74 (137–163)
1.70 (5'7")	58–65 (127–143)	60–69 (133–152)	64–76 (142–167)
1.73 (5'8")	60–66 (131–145)	62–71 (137–155)	66–78 (146–171)
1.75 (5'9")	61–68 (135–149)	64–72 (141–158)	68–80 (150–175)
1.78 (5'10")	63–69 (139–152)	66–73 (145–161)	70–81 (154–179)
1.80 (5'11")	65–70 (143–155)	68–75 (149–165)	72–83 (159–183)
1.83 (6")	67–72 (147–159)	70–77 (153–169)	74–85 (163–187)
1.85 (6'1")	69–75 (151–165)	71–80 (157–175)	76–86 (167–189)
1.88 (6'2')	70–76 (155–168)	73–81 (161–179)	78–89 (171–197)
1.90 (6'3")	72–79 (157–173)	75–84 (166–185)	80–92 (176–202)

Women

Height m (ft)	Small frame kg (lbs)	Medium frame kg (lbs)	Large frame kg (lbs)
1.50 (4'11")	42–51 (93–112)	44–55 (98–121)	48–57 (106–125)
1.52 (5')	44–52 (96–115)	46–57 (101–124)	49–58 (109–128)
1.55 (5'1")	45–54 (99–118)	47–58 (104–127)	51–59 (112–131)
1.57 (5'2")	46–55 (102–121)	49–60 (107–132)	52–61 (115–135)
1.60 (5'3")	48–56 (105–124)	50–62 (110–135)	54–63 (118–138)
1.63 (5'4")	49–58 (108–127)	51–63 (113–138)	55–65 (122–142)
1.65 (5'5")	50–59 (111–130)	53–64 (117–141)	57–66 (126–145)
1.68 (5'6")	52–60 (115–133)	55–66 (121–144)	59–67 (130–148)
1.70 (5'7")	54–62 (119–136)	57–67 (125–147)	61–69 (134–151)
1.73 (5'8")	56–63 (123–139)	58–68 (128–150)	62–71 (137–155)
1.75 (5'9")	58–64 (127–142)	60–69 (133–153)	64–73 (141–159)
1.78 (5'10")	59–66 (131–145)	62–71 (137–156)	66–75 (146–165)
1.80 (5'11")	61–68 (135–148)	64–72 (141–159)	68–77 (150–170)
1.83 (6')	63–69 (138–151)	65–74 (143–163)	69–79 (153–173)

Find your BMI 'score' on the chart below or see the box on page 26 for an explanation of how to calculate it exactly.

amount of muscle mass, but it is a more accurate measure of body fat than weight alone. It's based on a ratio of weight to height, so the first thing you need to do, since you already know your height in metres, is weigh yourself in kilograms. Don't guess, and for an accurate picture do it first

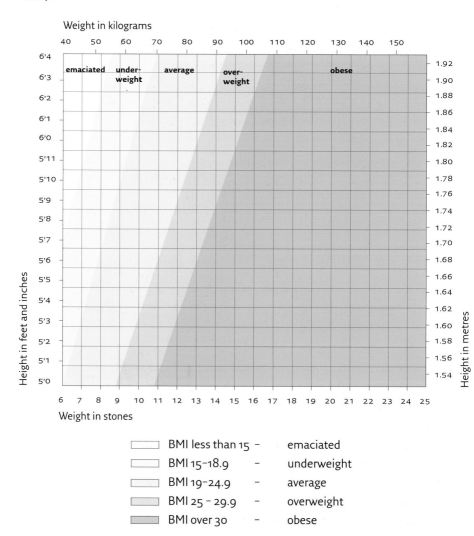

		BMI less than 15	–	emaciated
		BMI 15–18.9	–	underweight
		BMI 19–24.9	–	average
		BMI 25 – 29.9	–	overweight
		BMI over 30	–	obese

thing in the morning, after you've been to the loo but before getting dressed. Place your scales on a hard floor. (You'll find more about weighing yourself reliably in chapter 5.)

Using the BMI chart opposite, trace a line from your weight and another from your height. The point at which they intersect shows the range your BMI falls into.

If your BMI is below 15 or over 30, then you should see your doctor. But do remember that it is an average scale and doesn't differentiate by sex. There's a different BMI chart for children and young people under the age of 18. Athletes and pregnant women wouldn't get appropriate readings, and there's some ethnic variation, too. However, the BMI index can still give you useful guidelines.

Let's look at what the groups really mean.

• If your BMI is below 15, you are likely to be severely damaging your health because you are so underweight. You should certainly see your doctor, and you should actively try to put weight on.

• If your BMI is between 15 and 18.9, then you are classed as underweight and also need to put some weight on – you should be eating more to give your body the energy it needs.

• If your BMI is between 19 and 24.9, then you're a healthy weight. You are likely to be eating the right amount but remember that you still have to eat healthily. One thing – some authorities feel that this range is actually too broad, and that 24.9 is a little high. Try to avoid your BMI creeping upwards if you're at that end of the 'average' bracket.

• With a BMI of between 25 and 29.9, you're classed as being overweight. Your health would improve if you lost some weight, and you must try not to put any more on. Start taking more exercise, moderate what you eat, and aim for slow, steady and gentle weight loss.

• You're categorized as obese if your BMI is above 30, and you may well be putting a real strain on your health. Try to lose weight, but be careful to do so in a healthy way; you don't want to put additional pressure on your system with fad diets.

• There are two other gradations: from 35 to 39.9 and above 40. If you fall into either of these bands then your weight is very likely to be having a serious effect on your health and may well be shortening your life significantly. It is important to talk to your GP.

You can use BMI to give you a target weight, just as you can use a height and weight chart. Find your height on the BMI scale and trace the line until you are in the average group; now trace lines from both the beginning and end of that category up to the weight scale to see what you would have to weigh to fall into that group. You'll have quite a wide range.

must know

Waist to hip

Check your waist-to-hip ratio. Measure your waist at its narrowest point and your hips where they are widest, and divide the waist measurement by the hip one. If you are a man and you get 1.0 or above, or a woman who gets 0.85 or above, then you should take action; you need to get the ratio lower.

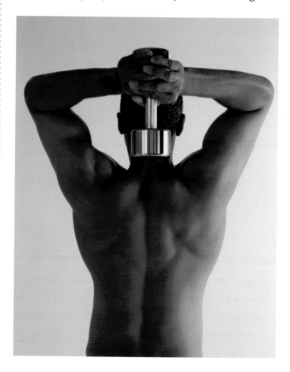

Muscle uses more energy than fat so it's worth increasing your muscle mass with a weight-training programme.

For example, if you were 1.68m tall (5ft 6in), your healthy weight would fall between 54 and 70kg (119 and 153 lbs). This broad range covers both men and women, and a man would normally have a higher BMI than a woman because of his (generally) greater muscle mass. But broad or not, you can use that range as a guide. If you are a woman who is 1.68m tall, head for somewhere in the middle of the range. A weight of 62kg would give you a healthy BMI of 22. If you currently weigh 80kg, you have 12kg to lose.

Work out how much you personally need to lose to get to what is a realistic target for you and double-check it against your height on the height and weight chart; together they can give you a relatively rounded picture, a good starting point.

You'll notice how wide the BMI range is if you look at both the male and female figures on the height and weight chart – the higher figure will generally appear on the men's part of the height and weight chart. This is why, if you're a woman, you shouldn't aim for the top end of the healthy BMI range except as a milestone on the way. Similarly, if you're a man the figure at the bottom end of the healthy BMI range would probably be too low.

How much should you eat?

Now we come to the method for calculating calorie intake which is favoured by many professionals. It's based on how much weight you have to lose, and you now have a realistic idea of that.

• If you're a woman with more than 19kg to lose, then you should be eating 1750 calories a day. If you have between 6.5 and 19kg to lose, eat 1500 calories. Eat 1250 calories a day if you have less than 6.5kg to lose.

must know

How big is your waist?

Carrying weight around the middle can indicate potential trouble. If you have a large waist – above 88cm (35in) for women and above 102cm (40in) for men – you're in the highest risk category for high blood pressure, heart disease and stroke. Talk to your GP about a diet and exercise programme.

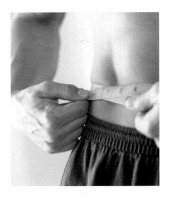

Find the point midway between your lowest rib and your hip bone, and measure there. Keep the tape snug but not tight – and don't breathe in.

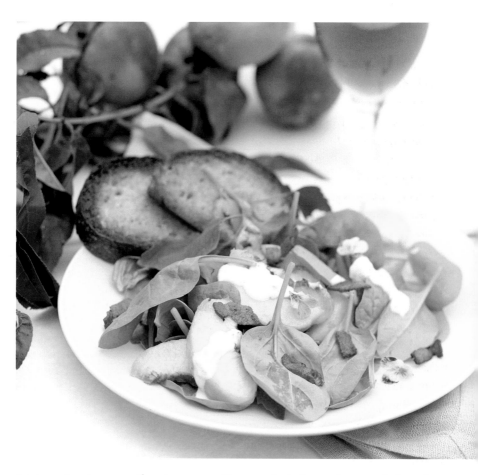

Salads need not be dull. Incorporate different colours, textures and flavours.

• If you're a man with over 19kg to lose, eat 2000 calories a day. If you're in the middle band, needing to lose between 6.5 and 19kg, eat 1750. If you've got less than 6.5kg to shift, eat 1500 calories.

These figures, for both men and women, assume that you're doing 30 minutes of aerobic exercise – a form of physical activity that makes you breathe faster – between three and five times a week. They should enable a gentle rate of weight loss of somewhere between 0.5 and 0.9kg a week; don't ever try to lose more weight than this. If you find that eating at these levels means the weight is falling off too fast, calm down. You may be eating too little, but it is equally likely that you lose a lot at the start and the rate will even out as time goes on.

Similarly, you may find that eating these quantities means the weight isn't coming off as quickly as you hoped. You may be being too ambitious; check that your goals are realistic. Another way of making sure that your target is reasonable is to think in terms of percentages – losing 1 per cent of your current body weight per week is absolutely fine, and will give you the best chance of keeping the weight off permanently. Less is fine, too, as long as the loss is consistent, so remind yourself how important it is for weight loss to be gradual. If there still seems to be a problem, double-check your calorie counting as something may be going adrift; make sure you're not forgetting between-meal snacks, or absent-minded nibbles, which is very easy to do. There's more on the practicalities of cutting calories in chapter 5.

Note: as you lose weight you'll have to adjust your calorie intake to reflect your new weight, so follow the guidelines above. Do not, under any circumstances, be tempted to go below 1000 calories. Eating at such a level for any length of time will have drastic effects on your health. Extreme dieting can very easily tip over into an eating disorder – it's a fine line anyway – so stop yourself if you're tempted.

Estimate how long your weight-loss goal should take to achieve at a rate of 0.5kg a week. There will be times when you slip or progress stalls but try to keep yourself on track overall. Now that you know what you are letting yourself in for, it's a good idea to look at motivation.

Motivating yourself

Dieting for a long period of time can seem daunting. The first thing to tell yourself is that it doesn't have to seem like a diet, and that you will accustom yourself to it remarkably quickly,

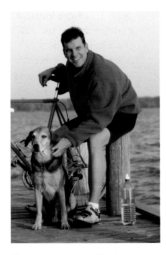

Dogs are a good motivator because they need to be walked whether you feel like it or not.

though it may not seem that way at first. The next thing to tell yourself is that the gentler the process, the more successful it will be. What you are doing is changing your life, and you can't really expect that to happen overnight. Here are some reasons for sticking with your diet.

It may be that you want to lose weight to benefit your appearance, but the real gain is in boosting your life expectancy and improving your all-round health. Looking better is really just the icing on the cake (though neither icing nor cake would actually be involved that often...). Remember that to succeed at changing anything you have to believe that change is important, and that you'll succeed in the end if you persist.

The health risks associated with being overweight or obese can be a powerful motivator rather than just something to worry about because they are something you can control, after all. These really are things you can change, and you're going to. Losing weight can significantly lower the risk.

Even small changes help. You can lower your blood pressure by losing as little as 10 per cent of your excess weight, and decrease the risk of potentially fatal conditions like stroke. If you lose weight the levels of triglyceride and cholesterol in your blood will drop, reducing your risk of cardiovascular disease. You'll be much less likely to develop type 2 diabetes if you get rid of your excess weight, and that can cause all sorts of problems including circulatory disorders which could eventually lead to limb amputation. You'll have less chance of developing osteoarthritis, and if you've already got it you'll find life much easier because you won't be putting so much strain on your joints or lower spine. You'll also be putting much less strain on your heart. You'll be less likely to have problems during surgery or anaesthesia and your recovery after operations can be quicker if you lose weight. In fact, if you are overweight surgery is sometimes delayed; this isn't some kind of moral judgement, it's simply that the risks associated with an operation may be too great – you are just more likely to develop complications during surgery. Then there's cancer. Being overweight or obese is a risk factor for many cancers, including colon, breast and bowel, the prostate in men, the uterus and cervix in women... There are some truly alarming statistics, but the good thing is that they all improve if you lose weight.

There are, of course, many other reasons, from practical ones, like wishing to restart a sport you used to enjoy, to social ones, like an important event (give yourself enough time if it's the latter; you don't want to put all the weight back on afterwards because you lost it too quickly). Whatever your reasons are, it is worth making a comprehensive list. Think about it for several days and write it down; hang on to it, as it can be useful later on.

It's also very important to think of what you are about to do as a lifestyle change, a fundamental alteration in the way you live your life, so...
• Tell yourself and believe that even the most long-standing habit or behaviour can be changed and you can do it.
• Don't try to be perfect all the time – use the 80:20 rule (see box, right) and be good most of the time.
• Don't dwell on dieting disasters of the past; they've got nothing to do with the present. Besides, failing

must know

The 80:20 rule

The dieter's version of the 80/20 principle is a little bit different to the scientist's. Use the 80:20 ratio to remind yourself that you don't have to be perfect 100 per cent of the time; 80 per cent will be fine. You can apply this 80:20 balance to other things, too – like the proportion of wholemeal to white bread. Go for being good enough, not impossibly ideal.

on a fad diet is no reflection on you anyway – it's a reflection of the inadequacy or stupidity of the diet.
• Finally, a single slip doesn't have to mean the end of your diet. Accept that it happened and move on.

Children

Concern is growing about the increase in childhood obesity. Current figures indicate that around 17 per cent of children in the West are obese – obese, not overweight, mind: seriously endangering their health. In some extreme cases this can even mean that they are likely to die before their parents. An obese adolescent is highly likely to become an obese adult, with all the associated risks. Everyone wants to be nice to their kids and give them what they like, by and large, but do be aware of the potential problems. It may sound obvious but, despite increasing publicity and efforts in schools, children don't necessarily realize the consequences of eating or drinking lots of things that are bad for them.

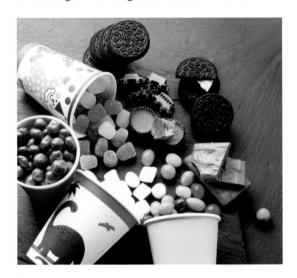

must know

Go easy on yourself

When you're dieting, one of the secrets of success is to make it as easy for yourself as you can. Don't put your willpower to impossible tests; you'll definitely weaken at some point because everyone does. So don't, for example, try and stick to low-calorie eating if you're being taken out for a birthday meal but plan for it instead, and don't keep packets of savoury snacks in the cupboard if you can't resist them. Set yourself up to succeed.

If you don't keep sweet treats in the house, children won't pester you for them quite so often.

Because of the wide variations in children's height and rate of growth, adult BMI scales don't apply to them. Paediatric BMI charts are available, and you should ask your doctor if you are concerned about a child or young person. Children go through growth spurts and can vary enormously, so do this before you consider taking action.

If there really is a problem, then the next step is to encourage activity. It is thought that the main reason for the alarming rise in childhood weight problems is the increase in the amount of time kids spend in front of televisions and computers. They are likely to graze on high-calorie food while watching TV or playing computer games, and on the whole they are much more sedentary than previous generations. Many children in the developed world today are a lot less active even than children were only a few years ago. Again, this can be changed and the effects can be dramatic. One recent study showed that in children whose TV and computer use was limited to an hour a day there were significant decreases in both weight and body fat.

Weight management is often the key to controlling children's weight, rather than formal dieting. Reducing or limiting junk food and high-calorie snacks is a vital part and can have spectacular rewards, and the more active children are, the less time they have to snack.

want to know more?

• If you are worried about a child's weight, look at the information available at the Institute of Child Heath website – www.ich.ucl.ac.uk.
• There are also helpful books, such as Karen Sullivan's *How to Help Your Overweight Child*, which has many useful ideas, especially on persuading children to eat healthy food.
• For information on how to put your new resolve into practice, check out chapter 4.

websites

• www.eatwell.gov.uk/ healthydiet/healthy weight
• www.nationaleating disorders.org
• www.eatright.org

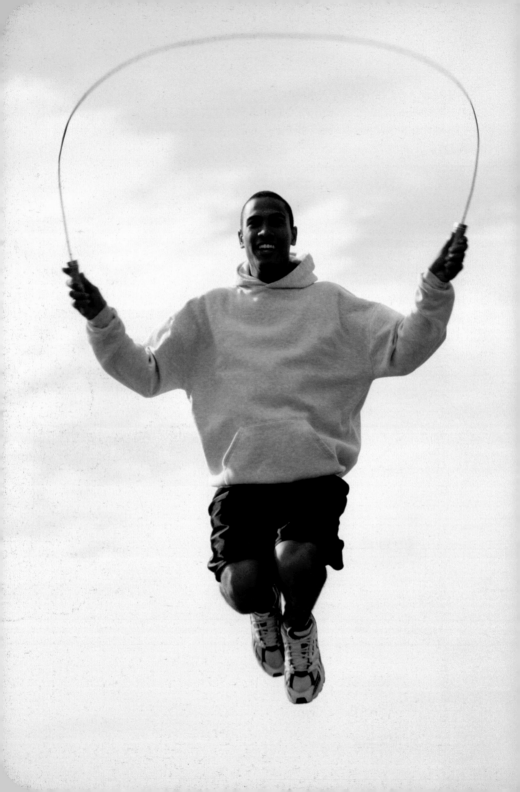

3 Improving energy out

Exercise is crucial for sustaining a long-term process of gradual weight loss and for preventing your lost weight from finding you again. Increasing overall physical activity is the best thing you can do to help maintain your new weight once you've got to where you want to be. Studies have shown very clearly that those people most likely to keep to their new weight following a diet are those who raise their levels of physical activity and exercise.

Improving energy out

Physical activity is an important part of any serious attempt to lose weight. Controlling what we eat is just one side of the equation: the other side is the energy we use. Exercise is not a substitute for dieting but the two work hand in hand.

must know

Sports drinks

Steer clear of sports drinks and watch out for anything labelled as 'high-energy', 'sports' or which claims to 'give you energy' - this actually means that it will give you calories, often lots of them, generally in the form of glucose.

First thoughts...

The body has a point at which it will defend its current weight, one at which losing more weight can be difficult. If you use more calories than you eat, at some point your body will automatically become more efficient at using those calories that it does ingest. This point – sometimes called its 'set point' – can be altered, but doing so permanently requires a long-term effort and a certain amount of retraining for your body. Eating more healthily is part of the picture, and increasing your level of physical activity can also help.

The first important thing to remember is that it's the overall level of physical activity that's important. Building muscle will ultimately improve your RMR, but just getting out of the car or off the sofa is where it starts. Increased activity really kicks in over the long haul.

Every activity you undertake burns calories, whether it's walking the dog, kicking a ball about with the children, reading or working out in the gym. In fact, some activities that you might automatically class as 'exercise', like doing an aerobics class, burn off relatively few calories, fewer than you'd imagine; you'll find a chart on page 42. Where formal exercise really helps is in building muscle mass, or helping

Before starting a running programme, get specialist advice on your technique. Incorrect moves can put strain on joints.

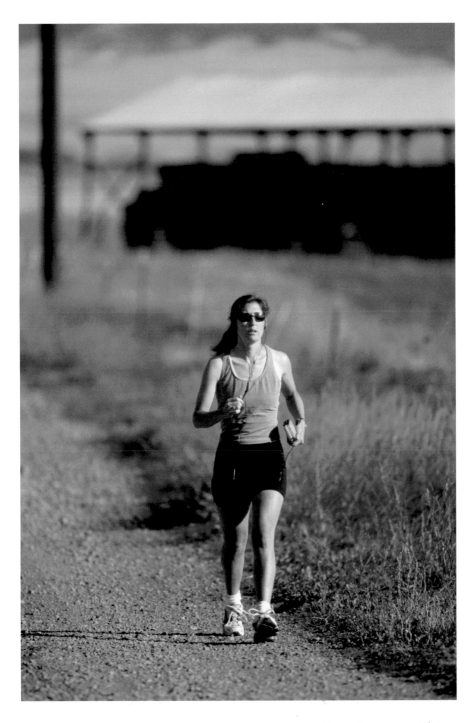

Number of calories burned in 30 minutes of activity (in relation to body weight)

Activity/exercise	50kg	55kg	60kg	65kg	70kg	75kg
Aerobics	155	170	185	200	225	250
Badminton	190	200	210	220	230	240
Basketball	310	350	390	430	470	500
Bowling	95	100	105	110	115	120
Canoeing	120	125	135	140	145	150
Carpentry	125	135	140	145	150	160
Cooking	70	75	80	85	90	95
Cycling	150	165	180	195	210	240
Dancing, moderate	115	120	130	135	140	150
Dancing, fast	300	310	320	330	340	350
Dish-washing	70	75	80	85	90	95
Dressing	40	40	45	45	50	50
Driving	50	55	60	65	70	75
Exercise, moderate	150	160	170	180	190	200
Exercise, fast	200	220	240	260	280	300
Football	275	300	325	350	375	400
Gardening	120	130	140	150	160	170
Golf, no cart	120	125	130	140	145	150
Golf, with cart	70	75	80	85	90	95
Handball	260	275	290	310	330	350
Hockey (field or ice)	300	310	320	330	340	350
Horseback-riding	130	140	150	160	170	180
Housework, active	100	105	110	120	125	135
Ironing	70	70	75	75	80	80
Jogging, light	225	235	245	255	265	275
Lacrosse	300	315	330	345	360	375
Office work	65	70	75	80	85	90
Painting (walls)	130	135	140	150	160	170
Piano playing	100	105	110	115	120	125
Reading	15	15	20	20	25	25
Rowing	325	350	375	400	425	450
Running, slow	290	315	345	375	405	435
Running, fast	375	415	450	490	525	550
Sewing	25	25	30	30	35	35
Singing	35	40	45	50	55	60
Sitting at rest	15	15	20	20	25	25
Skating, energetically	250	260	270	280	290	300
Skiing, energetically	250	260	270	280	290	300

Activity/exercise	50kg	55kg	60kg	65kg	70kg	75kg
Stair climbing	170	185	200	215	230	250
Sweeping floor	70	75	80	90	100	110
Swimming, slow	190	210	230	250	270	290
Swimming, fast	240	260	285	305	330	355
Tennis	165	180	195	215	230	245
Typing	85	90	95	100	105	110
Volleyball	170	185	200	215	230	250
Walking, moderately	105	115	125	135	145	155
Walking, fast	125	135	145	155	165	175
Writing	50	55	60	65	70	75

you to retain it. Resistance exercises, sometimes called anaerobic exercises – often using weights or hydraulics for muscles to pull against – are the best way of building muscle mass, but it doesn't have to be as agonizing as it sounds.

Here's a bit more motivation. Upping your levels of physical activity won't only help your diet; it will also improve your chances of living longer and being healthier all round. It has many of the same health benefits as losing excess weight – lowering the risk of heart disease, cancer, type 2 diabetes – but it also helps to build bone density, thereby helping to prevent osteoporosis and arthritis from developing (and it even seems to help to relieve some of the pain for those who already have arthritis). Best of all, perhaps, it reduces anxiety and depression – it really does improve your mood. And you don't have to spend hours in a sweaty, smelly gym, because brisk walking can give you many of the same benefits.

Before you begin

One word of warning – if you are overweight and are planning on increasing your exercise level, you must consult your doctor. This is especially important if you've not undertaken any exercise for some time, or if you're over 50, or both. You want

must know

Run for the money

Motivate yourself by
joining a money-raising
event. Many charities
organize fun runs,
either locally or
nationally, so check
with your favourite
good cause and raise
some money while
you're getting fitter.

to make sure there's no problem with the blood
supply to your heart, so get it checked out.

There are different sorts of exercise: aerobic
exercise and the resistance or anaerobic exercise
mentioned earlier. But first, and particularly
important if you're at all exercise- and sport-phobic,
think about incorporating more exercise into your
everyday routine. You may find it more helpful to
think of it as simple physical activity rather than
exercise – not quite so intimidating.

Everyday activity

It's all too easy to slip into a relatively sedentary
lifestyle, and you need to change the situation if it's
happened to you. If you drive or ride to work, use the
car to go shopping or take children to school, work
in an office sitting at a desk all day, and then come
home and flop in front of the television or computer,
you're essentially sedentary. It's insidious; you don't
really notice it happening. So think about your own
day. How much walking do you actually do? How
much moving around? It might be a lot less than you
think. Try wearing a pedometer to count your steps –
experts recommend that we get up to 10,000 each
day, so a couple of thousand isn't brilliantly high!

One of the things it's worth considering is how
much time you spend watching TV, and how long
you spend at the computer. There is a definite link
between spending lots of time on sedentary
activities and being overweight, which is particularly
clear in children. Try to cut this time down, and do
something active instead. Making gradual changes
is the key to success with activity levels as with so
many other things. You don't have to do everything

at once, and it's actually much better for you in the long term if you don't.

Working in the house and garden can easily be increased. Cleaning the house, washing the car, doing the garden – they are all forms of exercise; try ironing while watching TV as a starter. Decorating is great exercise (using a paint roller can be a good workout for your arms) so do it yourself instead of paying someone else. You may think you haven't got the time, but run a quick check on how long you spend just chilling out. Use some of that.

If you have children, get them involved; this can have far-reaching benefits as you are leading by example. Think a bit laterally; it doesn't have to be something sporty. Gardening is a good example. Encourage your children to grow something of their own, preferably something they can eat that grows quickly. A window box full of lettuce leaves is fairly speedy and may even get them eating their greens, and you can be out there with them, growing something of your own too. You would, after all, be picking up on a real trend: sales of vegetable seeds in the UK have just outstripped those of flower seeds for the first time since the Second World War and the 'dig for victory' campaign; allotment use is becoming fashionable and anyway home-grown veg is much nicer than anything you can buy in a supermarket.

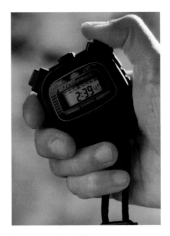

Some good-quality pedometers tell you the calories burned as well as the number of steps taken.

must know

Joining a gym

Unless money is no object, don't go mad and splash out on expensive gym membership immediately. There are many local authority gyms which provide similar equipment and classes, and which are much cheaper.

Walking

One of the simplest things you can do to boost your activity level is to walk more. When you're out, always use stairs rather than lifts or escalators. Park as far away from the entrance to the supermarket as you can. If you commute to work, get off your bus or

must know

Family walks

One of the advantages of walking is that you can involve the whole family. Children and young people may well enjoy the planning: www.walkingworld .com is a subscription website, but it's reasonably priced and you can find tips, download maps and see a photograph for over 3,000 walks. See also www.ramblers.org.uk and www.exodus.co.uk.

train a stop before you need to and walk the remaining distance instead. Walk the children to school instead of piling them into the car: good for you, good for them and even good for the environment. Wear your pedometer again and check the number of steps you take each day; it should have increased. Build on that figure gradually and aim for that goal of 10,000 steps during a single day.

But there's more to walking than that. Brisk walking can offer as many benefits as getting up early and jogging. One of the biggest studies of health and nutrition, the Nurses' Health Study in the USA, has demonstrated a very clear link between walking and preventing heart disease. Women who walked infrequently were much more likely to have a heart attack than those who walked briskly for an

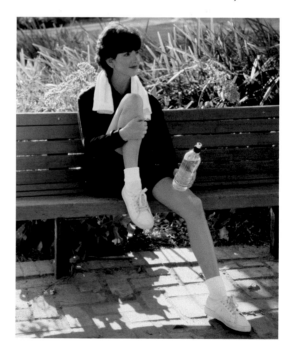

Don't forget to stay hydrated when you exercise. You may like to take a small towel if you are prone to sweating.

average of only three hours a week; they were less at risk of developing diabetes, too. When you consider that there are 168 hours in a week, that's not really very much – less than 2 per cent of your time.

Walking, of course, can be done anywhere, doesn't necessarily call for special equipment, doesn't have to involve paying joining fees or membership, and is quite safe. It's also very popular, so if you want to join a group, it's easy enough to find one. In the UK, walking is the most popular physical activity in which to participate, and there are extensive public rights of way to explore, but you don't have to live in the country to take it further.

Start exploring your local area; many cities have guided walks, so join one in yours. There are often suggested routes to explore on your own, but you don't even need that: there are few things more pleasant than wandering around a beautiful area. Many industrial cities have fascinating walks which explore their heritage, so visit your local tourist information centre and pick up leaflets.

If you're treating yourself to a city break abroad, then amble around the place you're visiting; you'll get a much better impression of it than you would if you just used public transport between tourist attractions. If you're uncertain about routes, then take a guided walking tour and retrace it later, exploring the enticing side streets that your tour guide bypassed.

Once you get into it, you can extend your walking and try a walking weekend in the country, maybe on the coast or in hills and woods. Or you can go a bit further, and look at walking weekends in Europe – there are many options once you start investigating.

must know

Walking snacks

If you're planning a long walk, pack your rucksack or backpack bearing your diet in mind – so no energy bars or Kendal Mint Cake. Instead take some unsalted nuts, dried fruit and a couple of apples or a banana – and don't forget to include a bottle of water.

If you enjoy walking, why not try some of the 'once in a lifetime' walks? There are companies that specialize in these, or you can arrange them yourself with a little research. Think about Peru's Inca Trail; the beautiful Milford Track in New Zealand; paths following Native American trails in the Grand Canyon; or even the gorgeous West Highland Way in Scotland. You need to be reasonably fit to undertake these, so make one of them an aim, a fantastic reward to head for. For even more motivation you could always join a charity challenge; China is a popular destination, as is South America.

Aerobic exercise

If you've got visions of aerobic exercise as a bunch of sweaty people going for 'the burn' in a hot local gym studio, think again. An aerobic exercise is any exercise that gets you breathing faster, that you can maintain continuously, that has a rhythmic element and uses large muscle groups. Walking can be an aerobic exercise, though you might not usually think about it in that way. Dancing is another aerobic exercise, as are skipping, running, swimming and cycling.

Join a salsa class or learn flamenco, go to your local pool or get your bike out. Cycling is a great way to exercise and keep your heart healthy but it does need to be done regularly. Take reasonable safety precautions and start slowly if you haven't done any for years; build up your stamina gradually. Moderate cycling is good; fast cycling, and cycling up hills, is even better.

Whatever you decide to do, proceed gradually. Start by having a quick swim a couple of days a week,

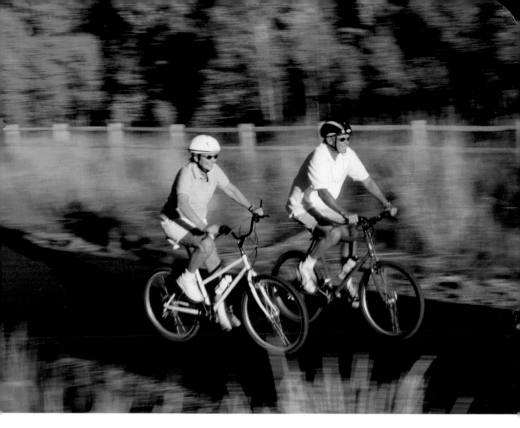

and build up. Always choose something you know you are likely to enjoy, and be realistic. If the thought of joining an exercise class makes your blood run cold, don't do it. If the only bellydancing group you can find is over an hour's journey away you won't stick with it, no matter how much you want to. Be practical.

Another tip is not to get stuck in a rut; make sure you do lots of different things. Swim a couple of times a week, take a dance class, do more walking: these are all relatively painless ways of increasing the amount of exercise your body gets. So is dancing along to lively, bouncy music in your own home, so let yourself go and try something different – check out mambo or Cuban rhythms, or catchy West African beats (see www.worldmusic.net).

Exercising with a friend means you can help to motivate each other.

must know

Monitor TV time

Most people watch television for at least two hours a day, many for longer. Can you honestly not afford 30 minutes to exercise twice a week? Once you start you'll find it easier.

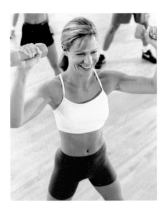

Get professional advice on the
correct way to use weights in
classic resistance exercises.

Resistance or anaerobic exercise

With resistance exercises, you're not exercising
continuously but going for short bursts of activity
followed by rests - weightlifting is a clear example.
Any exercise that makes muscles work against some
sort of resistance helps to build muscle mass. It
works best when you move slowly and try your best
to get the exercise right; not rushing is important.

Resistance exercise doesn't have to involve
weights, though; you can also work one part of your
body against another or use the floor to push
against. Press-ups are resistance exercises, as are
simple squats and leg lifts.

If you hate the idea of a class or gym, you can
develop a basic routine of your own, but do be
careful. If you try something and it hurts, stop
immediately. Only use recognized exercises - don't
try and make them up or you could damage yourself
- and do some research. Make sure, for example, you
think about balancing your exercise routine.

Here are a couple of basic exercises you could do
in your own home as a starter.

• For a basic squat, stand with your feet a little more
than hip-width apart. Extend your arms in front of
you and clasp your hands together. Now lower your
bottom as though you were going to sit down, hold
for one breath and push yourself back up. Repeat,
slowly and gently. Your weight should be on the back
part of your feet - test by lifting your toes.
• For a basic front raise you'll need two small bottles
of water or two 400g tins of beans. Have your legs in
the same position but keep you knees 'soft' (i.e.
don't lock them). Hold your water bottles or tins by

the sides of your body with your palms facing downwards and slowly raise your arms in front of you, keeping them straight, until they are at chest or shoulder height. Hold for a couple of beats, then go back to the start position and repeat.

Classes

Exercise classes might be less threatening than you imagine. Most people there tend to concentrate on what they should be doing rather than on other people in the class, and not all gyms are intimidating places. A traditional yoga class could be a good place to start; yoga attracts people of all ages and shapes, and a good teacher will make you feel welcome. Many Pilates groups are similarly friendly.

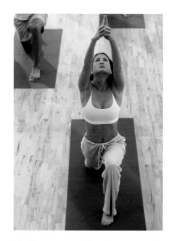

Finding a sympathetic exercise class may be easier than you think.

If you want to be more adventurous, boxercise – using moves normally found in boxing to work your lungs and heart – is fantastic for relieving stress, and you can find variations on traditional favourites, like Latin Step, a step class done with fab Latin music and moves. Shop around before ruling anything out.

A few more words of warning

Before doing any serious exercise there are some things everyone should consider. Remember you should talk to your GP if you are contemplating exercise for the first time in years or if you are overweight. Don't put your health at risk in your quest to get healthy. Do get yourself checked out and always build up gradually.

Think about any special equipment or clothing you need. This means items like cycle helmets and it also means making sure that any footwear fits properly. Sports or walking shoes should be tried on when

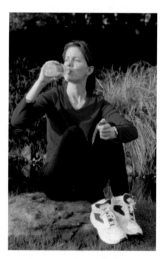

Don't push yourself too far. Rest at regular intervals when you feel you need to.

your feet are at their most swollen, probably in the afternoon or evening. Try a size bigger than your normal shoe size, and in the case of trainers, you should probably have more than one pair as they can get disgusting quickly. It's not just the smell; fungus can grow in overused trainers. Always make sure they dry out between sessions to help prevent this.

Women should wear a good sports bra – a bad one or your ordinary bra can affect your breathing as well as being painful, and not having sufficient support can lead to permanent sagging.

Warm up properly because not doing so makes it more likely that you will injure yourself. Start with small movements and increase them gradually. Marching on the spot is one simple suggestion, and so is arm circling. Spend time warming up first, and do some stretching afterwards.

Watch out for bad habits, either your own or those inherent in any sport you may take up. Tennis and golf are very one-sided, for example, and Pilates-style exercises are often recommended to help golfers correct that tendency.

Look out for any such habits you may be developing, and try to balance every workout accordingly. If you focus on one muscle or group of muscles, then it's important to work the opposing group of muscles to the same extent. While you can figure this out for yourself to some degree, it is probably best to seek advice.

Finally, remember that you will need liquid so don't forget to drink. Whatever you are doing, keep a bottle of water handy. You must keep yourself hydrated, but try not to take in extra calories at the same time.

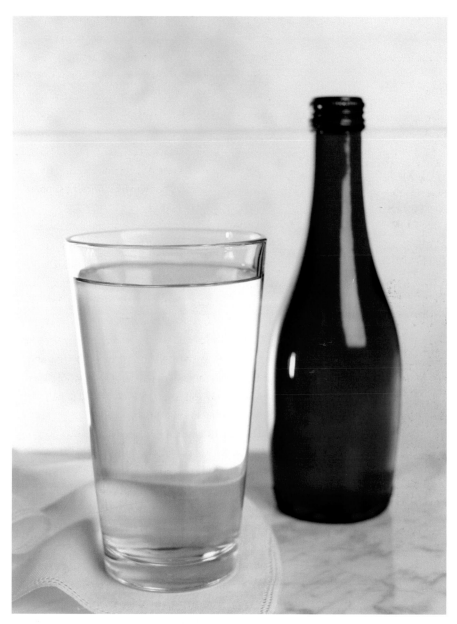

Try to drink about 2.25 litres of liquid a
day. The best choice is plain water.

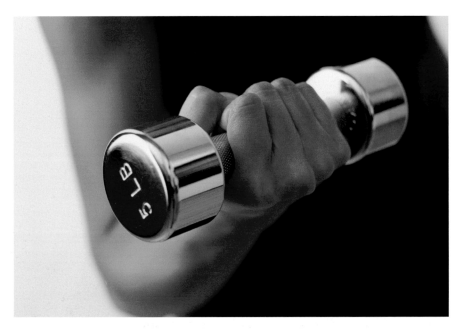

To build muscle strength do a few repetitions of each exercise with the heaviest weight you can manage comfortably.

Everyday exercise

If you have the sort of job where you spend your day sitting behind a desk, you may think there isn't a lot you can do to increase your activity while at work. However, once you begin to become naturally more active, you'll find plenty of things.

First of all, remember that the advice about walking more in a day doesn't just apply to getting to and from work. You could clock up several thousand extra steps by using the stairs in your office instead of taking the lifts and escalators. Give yourself excuses to travel to a different floor several times during the day. Use a loo on a different floor, or go to visit colleagues rather than emailing or phoning them. Stand up to talk on the telephone. Or try to stretch for things actively – put them just out of reach so you have no choice. And stretch down to pick up light things, like sheets of paper, from the floor while keeping your legs straight. Use your breaks to do a little walking, or find a convenient place to do a few surreptitious exercises. Physical activity can be incorporated into all kinds of tasks once you start thinking about it.

Watch your posture while you're at work. Stand up straight, with your shoulders back, and you will instantly look much thinner than if you slouch. Try to hold your stomach in quite tightly throughout the day; this is what is known as 'doing an all-day sit-up' and is one of the key elements of Pilates workouts. More technically, what you are doing is pulling in your abdominal muscles to about 75 per cent tension. Imagine you are walking around in a bikini or swimming trunks, which should help you to hold the correct muscles.

If you think your posture needs help, for example if you are prone to back pain, it's worth learning the Alexander Technique. To find a qualified teacher, go to www.stat.org.uk.

Here are some suggestions for little exercises that are quite easy to do at work, even at your desk. If anyone catches you, just explain that you are getting fit for a charity fun event, and that you'll be looking for their support (and sponsorship) later. (In fact, it's an extremely good idea to give yourself some public motivation by signing up for a charity event and getting all your work colleagues to sponsor you. It's much harder to pull out when everyone has signed your sponsorship form.)

• To loosen your shoulders, which can get hunched if you sit at a computer all day, do this simple stretch. Sit forward in your chair and link your hands behind your back; move your elbows back until you can feel your shoulder blades pulling together. Hold for 30 seconds and repeat.

• And if your neck gets stiff, try this. Sit up straight, then slowly lower your chin to your chest, return to the upright position and stretch gently. Without dropping your chin, turn your head to each side and repeat ten times.

• Bicep curls, which work the front of the arm, can be fairly inconspicuous if you have a bit of privacy. Hold a couple of small bottles of water by your sides, palms facing downwards as in the

must know

Gardening

Gardening can be a great form of exercise. There's lots of advice online, whether you have a window box or a huge plot. Try www.crocus. co.uk as a good place to begin.

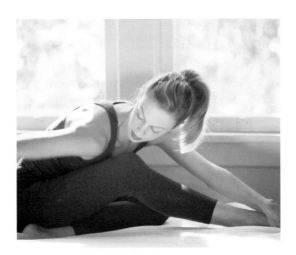

Stretching exercises keep your muscles long and supple.

Listening to music as you exercise makes the time pass more quickly.

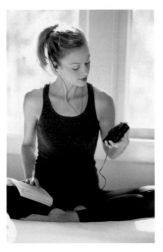

basic front raise on page 50. Keep your body as straight as possible and curl your hands upwards towards your shoulders, keeping your elbows close to your body. Slowly return to the start position.

• Calf lifts are good for your legs and, more generally, for your balance. Stand with your feet on the edge of a low step – if you have no access to a step for this one, save it for home – and let your heels drop below the level of the step. You may find it helpful to place your hands on your hips. Then rise up on to your toes, hold and repeat. Balancing may be a bit difficult at first, but it soon becomes easier.

You can always improvise exercise at home, too; you don't have to get down on the floor and do press-ups. Try running on the spot during the trailers or ad breaks on TV, do simple bicep curls (bending your elbow to raise the weight up to your shoulder) using 400g tins of tomatoes or beans, and use the bottom of the stairs for step-ups and calf lifts. If you want to get an exercise bike, check out eBay and your local charity shops for secondhand ones.

As a final encouragement, remind yourself of all the benefits of exercise:

• you'll find it easier to keep your weight down
• it will be better for your heart, your blood pressure, your cholesterol...
• you'll be less likely to develop type 2 diabetes as you're improving the way your body deals with glucose and insulin (muscle is just better at it)
• there'll be a reduced chance of you developing osteoporosis
• you'll be more supple and flexible, and less stressed
• and don't forget that doing some form of physical activity will cheer you up, lifting your mood.

In brief, doing more will help you to feel good, prevent the weight you lose from returning and keep you healthier. Just don't reward yourself with food. It has to be worth it.

want to know more?

• For more information on calories that can be burnt off during exercise, see www.fitnessonline.com/tools/calories.
• To remind yourself about why doing more is a good idea, go back to chapter 1.
• Get sensible information about exercise from books like Joanna Hall's *The Exercise Bible*.

websites

• www.eatwell.gov.uk/healthydiet/healthyweight/caloriecalculator – for calorie expenditure by exercise
• www.pedometers.co.uk, who also have compasses and other useful equipment for serious walkers.

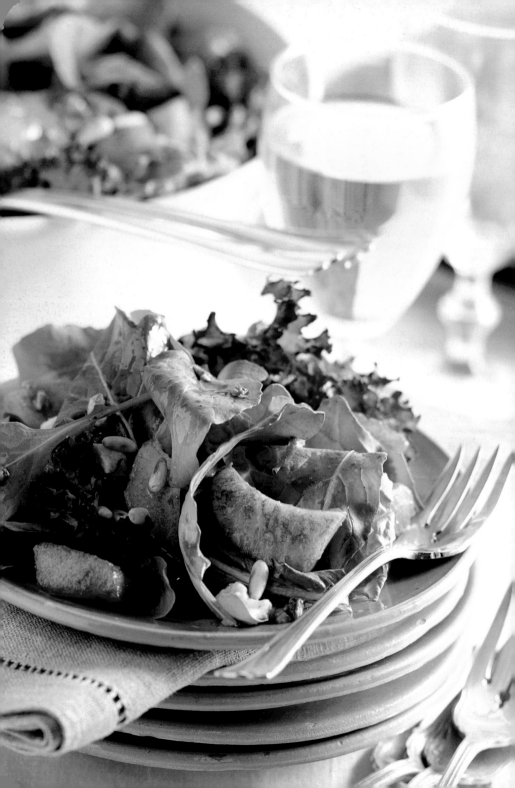

4 Improving energy in

There have always been a couple of problems associated with calorie counting, connected to the freedom it gives you. Theoretically you could eat whatever you wanted as long as you stayed below a certain number of calories per day, but your diet might not be healthy enough. If you want to change what you weigh, you really need to change what you eat, and not just reduce the quantities.

Improving energy in

If you carry on eating in the way you always have but cut back on calories, you may not get the nutrients your body requires. Without making fundamental changes to your diet, it may be difficult to keep the weight off when you achieve your target.

must know

Media scare stories

There are always stories about food and diet in the media, and it's important to keep a cool head. Don't believe everything you read, but get hold of a good, balanced guide like *Nutrition for Dummies* by Nigel Denby, Sue Baic and Carol Ann Rinzler.

Why did you gain weight?

If someone has gained weight, there's a good chance they've been eating unhealthily. Modern diets are often exceptionally high in sugary or fatty foods anyway – the very things that make it easy to put weight on. Most experts agree that the increasing consumption of food high in sugar and fat is directly tied to the increasing incidence of overweight and obesity. Another factor is that most people nowadays eat a lot of refined products – like white bread and other items made from white flour – and processed food. These can be low in essential nutrients.

Fortunately it doesn't have to be too painful to make changes for the better, and if you find it difficult remind yourself of the reasons why you're doing it. You may want to reread the list of reasons you made (described in chapter 2), or write some down now. Don't forget that change can, in fact should, be gradual; you don't have to do everything at once. However, in two particular areas you should make every effort to change as soon as possible, as they can both have almost immediate effects.

The first area is 'junk food', whether you're tempted by fast food or high-sugar and high-fat snacks. The more of those you eliminate from your diet, the better. Your calorie intake will go down automatically, as will the amount of saturated fat you are eating, which can only do you good.

The second is ready meals and convenience food. Processed food contains many ingredients you wouldn't normally cook with – for instance, xanthan gum, sodium stearoyl-2-lactylate, tartrazine – and may be so processed that essential ingredients are lacking. Highly processed food generally tends to have lost its vitamins and fibre, and other additives are put in to compensate. Some have a useful role while others are cosmetic, but the fact remains that if you cook for yourself you just won't need to break out the sodium stearoyl-2-lactylate.

Many ready meals have higher sugar and fat levels than the home-cooked equivalent, and use lots of refined products – just what you want to avoid if you're trying to lose weight. There are strategies you can adopt for saving time when you need a quick meal; check out chapter 5. It's fine to have the occasional ready meal, just don't base your diet around them. Remember 80:20 and be good 80 per cent of the time. Nobody's perfect!

must know

Shop locally

Finding good food locally is getting easier. Food co-ops are appearing in some areas, providing fresh vegetables and seasonal fruits, and farmers' markets are much more common. Try www.farmers markets.net and www.farma.org.uk to see what's in your area.

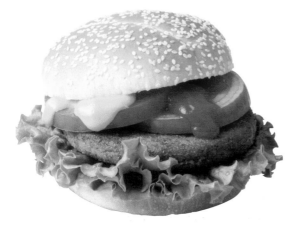

Removing the top half of the bun from your burger can save over 80 calories.

What makes up a healthy diet?

Food contains macronutrients – carbohydrates, proteins, fats – which the body needs in large quantities for energy, growth and development. It also needs large amounts of fibre, and the micronutrients which all food contains in much smaller amounts – vitamins and minerals. Micronutrients are used by the body in tiny quantities, but they are vital if it is going to function normally. Despite what some fad diets may say, macro- and micronutrients are all necessary.

Most food contains some or all of these in varying propor-tions; wholemeal bread, for instance, is generally thought of as a carbohydrate and so it is, but it also has significant amounts of protein, fat and fibre as well as vitamins and minerals. Vegetables and fruit are a great source of carbs – an apple is almost entirely carbohydrate though most of us would think of bread as a carb before we came up with apples – and both salmon and steak are a mixture of protein and fat. It is very important to eat a diet which balances food types. We all need liquids too, of course.

A good balance

Getting the balance right is not as difficult as it may seem, and there is no need to get bogged down. There are food pyramids and pie charts which can help, and there are also various official guides. Essentially you have to bear in mind a few simple proportions, because getting things roughly right in relation to each other is what you're aiming at.

Current government guidelines advise that our calories come from the following:
• carbohydrate: 47–50 per cent minimum
• protein: up to 15 per cent
• fat: 30–35 per cent maximum
• and you can add in alcohol, if you wish, but not more than 5 per cent.

It's not completely perfect – the World Health Organization and most experts recommend a maximum of 30 per cent fat – but it's a good start because of the flexibility it offers. You may well want to eat less fat, but remember that fat isn't just oil or butter or an ingredient in processed food: eggs, for example, are 61 per cent fat. Adding more carbs in the form of vegetables or fruit would be fine, but you should be wary of getting most of your carbs from white bread, pasta and rice. And percentages aren't that easy to use in practice.

Many diets suggest the image of a plate to help, and that can be more user-friendly. Cover half the plate with vegetables, a quarter with protein and the other quarter with starchy carbs like potatoes, pasta or rice, preferably whole grains. That will give you an idea of what you're aiming at. There are some quick practical tips for eating more healthily all round at the end of the chapter. Before that, let's look at the nutrients our bodies need.

Carbohydrates

Carbs are the basis of a healthy diet. They are usually found in grain products like bread or pasta, rice, fruits, vegetables, beans and pulses, and in dairy products. A low-fat yoghurt has more carbohydrate than it has protein or fat. During digestion, carbs are broken down into simple sugars like glucose.

It is important to choose the carbs that are best for you, and this choice is the basis of all the GI and GL diets – but it's relevant for everyone seeking to lose weight or improve their diet, or both. The glycaemic index (GI) groups foods according to the speed at which the sugar they contain is released into the bloodstream, and can be extremely useful when you're calorie counting. Opting for foods low on the GI or GL scales (GL means glycaemic load, the GI modified to take into account realistic portion sizes), keeps blood-sugar levels steady, avoiding spikes and sudden falls. This ensures that you'll feel full for longer. There can be quite a difference between the rate at which low

The glucose process

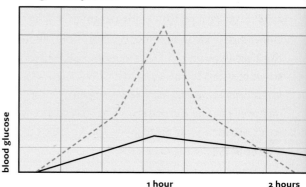

blood glucose

- - - - high GI food

—— low GI food

1 hour   2 hours

must know

Sardines

Canned sardines are a great source of calcium because you eat the bones, but go for those which are canned in spring water or tomato sauce rather than oil. Check labels across brands as some tomato sauces are quite high in calories.

and high GI carbs affect your body; low GI foods release glucose over several hours rather than instantly.

Generally, the carb-based foods to choose contain 'complex' carbs as opposed to the 'simple' carbs which have an almost-instant impact. Try to eat whole grains, and products made from them. Avoid white bread as you'll get much more satisfaction – and slightly fewer calories – from a similar quantity of wholemeal. Go for brown rice and try wholemeal pasta. Generally avoid refined-grain products; even if they are labelled 'fortified', you're still going to be better off with the whole-grain equivalent.

Low-GI food usually has more fibre, is less processed and lower in sugar than refined versions. As a quick guide, the sweeter something tastes, the more likely it is to have a swift effect on your blood sugar. Fibre can slow down the release of glucose so foods like whole grains, beans, most vegetables and fruit eaten with its skin are all better for you than refined grains, peeled potatoes (though they're not great even with the skin, because of the starch they contain, which is absorbed quickly) and fruit juice.

Whole grains

All processed grains, whatever they are, have been stripped of their outer coating, which is the part that has a high fibre content. However, where a GI diet would ban something like risotto rice completely, you can eat it when you are calorie counting – just don't rely on refined grains like that too often. Think 80:20 and balance it out. Oats are an excellent grain to choose and porridge at breakfast can see you through to lunchtime with no hunger problems. However, it is best to avoid heavily processed porridge oats; you don't need 'easy cook' anyway as porridge can only take about 5–10 minutes, and you may be able to find some with extra bran, which is nuttier and more flavoursome. Quinoa grains have recently become more popular, largely because they are one of the few complete plant sources of protein.

Vegetables and fruit

The UK's 'five-a-day' campaign highlighted the benefits of eating more fruit and vegetables, which is one of the best ways of improving your health. It really does work. One of the latest pieces of research shows that you can cut your risk of stroke by 11 per cent if you eat your five a day. If you eat more than the recommended five, your risk can go down by 26 per cent. There's the added benefit that many fruits and vegetables are either moderate or low in calories so they can fill you up without fattening you up.

Five portions a day are supposed to be a minimum, but even so many people don't get anything like that. Part of the reason may be some confusion about what constitutes a portion. Each of the following examples would make up one of your 'five':

must know

Steak

The less you cook a steak, the more fat it retains. A rare steak, originally weighing the same as a well-done steak, would cost you an extra 50 calories.

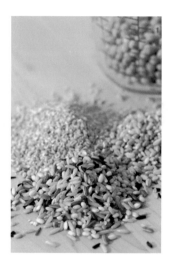

Grains are a great source of B vitamins, calcium, potassium and phosphorus. Go for whole grains when you can.

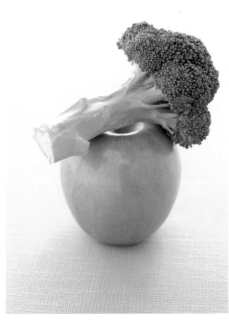

Eating more fruit and vegetables is one of the easiest ways of preventing disease and improving your health.

• one medium tomato
• an apple or pear
• a bowl of salad leaves
• 80g cherries – 14 should be about right
• a 100g slice of melon
• three small apricots or two plums
• two to three tablespoons of cooked vegetables (three for green veg, two for root vegetables and small ones like peas)
• half a grapefruit
• three tablespoons of fruit purée or tinned fruit (but watch out for the calories in tinned fruits and never buy them in syrup)
• three to four tablespoons of cooked lentils
• a handful – about 40g – of dried fruit
• 150ml of pure fruit juice.

Pulses and dried fruit can only be counted once, no matter how many portions you eat, and the same applies to fruit juice, though it would be better to eat the whole fruit. Potatoes don't count at all because they are so starchy.

Vegetables and fruits are great sources of micronutrients and some have been labelled 'superfoods' because they contain protective substances known as phytochemicals. These have all sorts of benefits, including blocking the activity of carcinogens (substances that can cause cancer). More is being discovered about them all the time, and antioxidants (see box on page 68), in particular, have had a lot of attention. One thing is certain – eating more fruit and veg can only help you.

Increasing fruit intake is easy because it's such a convenient snack. A mandarin orange is one portion, and only about 30 calories. Bananas are a good source of dietary fibre, and contain respectable amounts of vitamins A and C. They are higher in calories than most fresh fruit, but even so a small one might only be 55 calories. The classic snack for anyone on a diet is an apple, about 50 calories for a small one. They're also high in fibre, easy to transport and convenient to eat – plus they taste good. It is worth thinking about choosing organic, though, because of the large quantities of chemicals that are often used in conventional orchards. Substitute fruit for mid-morning biscuits (70 calories at least for a single digestive) and the chocolate bar which keeps you going until you get home, and you're benefiting both your weight-loss diet and your health. Fresh fruit is also the ideal dessert; just don't cover it in cream.

Some types of vegetables make great snacks – raw carrots, celery sticks and spring onions are handy ones. Increase the quantity of vegetables you consume with a main course (but not more potatoes) and be wise about cooking methods and sauces. You wouldn't get many calorie benefits from lots of deep-fried onion rings or a huge portion of carrots drowning in melted butter. Always include vegetables in sandwiches – tomatoes, cucumber, raw onion rings and a great handful of lettuce, for instance.

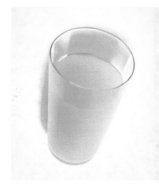

Fresh orange juice can count as one of your five-a-day but you'll get extra benefits from eating the whole fruit.

Pulses

Beans, dried peas and lentils are all pulses, and there are many types with different tastes and textures. They are important because they are great sources of complex carbs and protein as well as fibre. As you'd expect, they have a low GI, and because they are so filling a small quantity in terms of calories can be very satisfying. They are cheap too, especially if you buy them dried, and cans are a useful standby. Some people find beans hard to digest but they are too valuable a food source, and just too useful if you're calorie counting, to be ignored completely. Make sure you always rinse tinned beans: don't ever cook dried ones in their soaking water (see box on page 69) or add salt to the water you do cook them in. Tinned baked beans can be an

excellent emergency food, but as with all convenience foods you need to read the label. They may
well be high in salt and sugar, and may also contain
more calories than you'd expect.

Fibre
Everyone needs dietary fibre for a healthy digestive
system and most of us don't eat enough. When you're
dieting, fibre has many advantages: it makes food
take longer to eat and fills you up for longer once it's
been eaten. Fibre slows down the passage of food
through the digestive system and slows the absorption
of glucose into the bloodstream. Simply changing to
whole-grain products will painlessly increase your
consumption of fibre, and so will eating more fruit
and vegetables. Plant foods are the only source of
dietary fibre.

   If you're not used to eating foods that contain
decent amounts of fibre you may find it best to
change gradually, but don't be in any doubt that
change is desirable. The big EPIC study (EPIC stands
for European Protective Investigation of Cancer) has
shown that doubling your fibre intake halves your
risk of colon cancer. On a less dramatic level, it also
reduces any problems with constipation, which can
bedevil those diets that restrict carbs. There is one
other thing to bear in mind about fibre – be sure to
drink plenty of water to balance the water that fibre
absorbs.

Protein
Eating enough protein is essential for growth and
development, for maintaining and repairing the cells
of the body and for regulating its functions, among

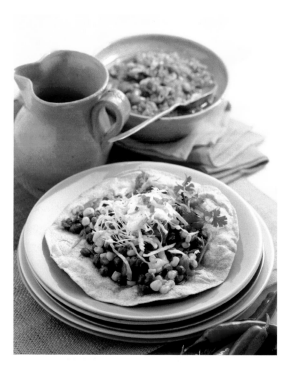

Pulses are low in fat, high in fibre and rich in vitamins and minerals. When eaten with grains, like this tortilla, they provide complete proteins too.

other things. Protein is broken down during digestion into amino acids and then absorbed into the bloodstream, and these amino acids are divided into two kinds, non-essential and essential. Non-essential amino acids can be made in the body; essential amino acids cannot be created by the body and must be obtained from food. There are nine essential ones.

Though protein deficiency is uncommon in the developed world, it does sometimes occur in dieters and vegetarians, so ensure that you are eating enough. Animal proteins contain all the essential amino acids, and so do quinoa, soya beans and products derived from soya like soya milk and tofu. Those are great for vegetarians, as well as everyone

must know

Serving veg

Vegetables are great for dieters, but there are pitfalls. As a simple shortcut, never eat vegetables with creamy sauces, ones that are covered in melted butter, anything in batter, or anything fried.

else, but if you are vegetarian you should also make certain that you're eating a combination of other plant proteins. That will have the same effect as eating 'complete', often animal-derived protein.

Meat, poultry and fish are good sources of complete protein, together with eggs and dairy products. Lentils, beans and dried peas are good plant sources, as are seeds and nuts. Unfortunately, nuts are very high in calories and fat, so you need to watch how many you eat.

This is the real reason why dieters can become deficient in protein - many of the good sources are high in fat, especially saturated fat, and are therefore high in calories. While it is important to bear this in mind, protein foods should not be avoided.

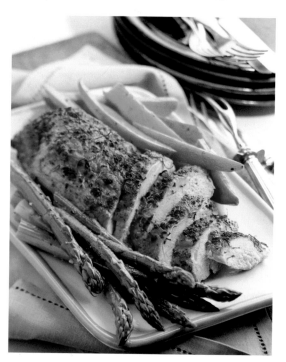

Turkey is a great choice for dieters. It's low in fat - but high in B vitamins, protein and selenium.

Eggs

There's no reason whatever to exclude eggs from your diet, even though they have been on the receiving end of some bad publicity. In some circumstances – if you are feeding small children, pregnant women or elderly people – you may be advised to be careful about raw or undercooked eggs; otherwise it would be a shame to miss out. For relatively few calories (78 for a medium one), eggs are a great source of protein. They contain all the essential amino acids in the correct proportions, and have significant quantities of micronutrients, including iron. Don't exclude eggs because of their cholesterol content, either. High levels of saturated fat have been shown to be far more significant in raising blood cholesterol. An egg a day is fine for most people.

Meat, poultry and fish

The general advice here is to moderate your intake of red meat, making sure that most visible fat is removed. Go for the leanest cuts possible and cook them in a healthy way, grilling or roasting on a rack so fat drips down. Reducing portion sizes also helps. Stir-frying can be good; lean meat tastes best in a stir-fry, and a little goes a long way. The leanest red meats are beef rump, fillet steak and topside, pork fillet and loin steaks, and game like venison. Watch out for the fat content of mince and avoid processed meat products like sausages and salami.

When cooking poultry, always remove the skin; white meat is lower in fat and calories. Again always grill poultry or roast it on a rack, and the best choices are chicken and turkey. Organic may be particularly

must know

Potatoes

Potatoes will affect your blood-sugar levels no matter how they are cooked; the best bet is boiled new ones. Spuds can also be deceptively heavy, and there can be a massive 230 calorie difference between a medium – 180g – baked potato and a large – 350g – one.

worth it here; intensively reared birds are often fed growth promoters and antibiotics.

Fish is a fantastic addition to the diet – in fact, it is recommended that it is eaten at least twice a week. It's a good source of protein and is low in fat, especially saturates. Oily fish – cold-water fish like salmon, tuna, herring and mackerel – are high in beneficial fats and shellfish is low in both fat and calories.

Dairy products

Milk and its derivatives are excellent from the nutrition point of view – generally – but they do contain a lot of fat, and are high in saturated fat, the one you really should try and cut down on (see page 76). It is best to try and get used to low-fat versions. Don't eliminate dairy products completely because your body needs the calcium they provide. If it doesn't get enough calcium from food, it will draw on its reserve stock – your bones – which can lead to osteoporosis. To maintain bone density, try not to cut down on dairy products too much.

Fortunately it is quite easy to get used to lower-fat versions. The best thing to do is, once again, adapt gradually. If you find something – like low-fat cheese, for instance – really unpalatable, then cut back on the quantity you eat instead. Don't do that with everything, however, or you'll soon be lacking calcium. With milk, go from full-cream milk to semi-skimmed and then to skimmed. You could even mix whole milk and semi-skimmed at first, gently increasing the proportion of the latter, but whatever you do, end up at skimmed. After a while, you'll even notice that full-cream milk tastes unpleasantly rich and fatty.

Low-fat plain yoghurt and no-fat Greek yoghurt are invaluable, but watch out for low-fat fruit yoghurts. They can often be higher in calories because sugar is added to replace the fat; it is better to add fruit to low-fat natural yoghurt yourself. Low-fat crème fraîche is a great substitute for cream and is also heat stable, so you can cook with it.

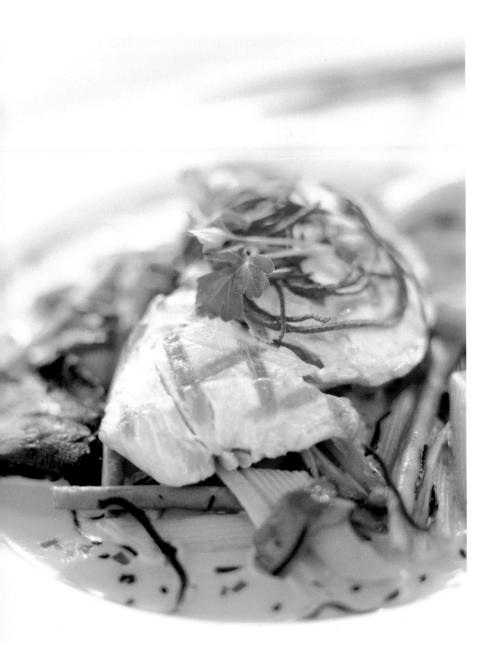

Fish has many health benefits and can be cooked quickly.

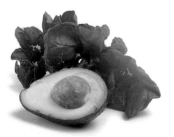

**Be careful what you serve with
avocado; it's high in calories
already.**

Not all cheeses are the same so choose those
lower in fat and calories if you really cannot tolerate
low-fat cheese. Watch out for the salt content of
cheeses as well.

Fats

Many dieters demonize fat, but some fat is necessary
for your body to function properly. It's an important
source of energy, the most concentrated one
available: 1g of fat provides 9 calories while 1g of
protein or carbohydrate provides 4 calories. It also
has other roles, making it possible for your body to
maintain a constant temperature, for instance. Not
all fats are the same, however, and most of us eat
too much of the wrong kind. A good first move is to
cut back on fat intake all round – it will help your
calorie counting, and it's vital for your health too.

There is another thing that makes dieters wary of
fat. Fat is broken down by digestion into fatty acids
and glycerol. Your body burns the energy from carbs
and proteins first and stores any excess fatty acids
and glycerol as fat. This has led people – including
many researchers – to believe that low-fat diets are
best. However, there is growing, serious evidence
that they don't work, that the fat in your diet doesn't
have to make you fat. If you eat more calories than
you use regardless of where they come from, you'll
gain weight. Fats have a vital role in keeping you
healthy, so it can be harmful to cut back on them all.

'Good' fats

Unsaturated fats are the healthy ones. They fall
into two categories: monounsaturated fats and
polyunsaturated fats.

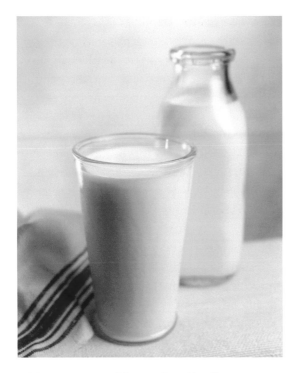

Get used to skimmed milk – dairy products are a vital source of calcium, so don't be tempted to cut them out.

Monounsaturated fats are found in olive, groundnut and rapeseed oils, spreads made from those oils, and walnuts and avocados. These have a positive effect on cholesterol levels.

There are two main types of polyunsaturated fats. These are known as essential fatty acids because they cannot be made by the body; they have to come from the diet. Omega-3 polyunsaturated fats are found in cold-water fish like mackerel, herring, salmon, tuna and sardines; in linseed, wheatgerm, sesame seeds, soya beans, the eggs of grain-fed chickens and in evening primrose oil; also in olive and rapeseed oils. Among other things, they play a part in regulating blood pressure and are essential for the normal functioning of the brain. Omega-6 polyunsaturated fats are present in vegetable, sunflower and corn oils, soya margarines and sunflower spreads. They are essential for cell growth and for keeping your immune system functioning. There's generally no need to deliberately increase the quantity of these, as most of us can get enough in a normal healthy diet. In fact, if you habitually use something like sunflower oil, it might be worth changing to rapeseed or olive – you'll still be getting enough omega-6 from other sources, but you'll be boosting your omega-3 and monounsaturates.

Fats to avoid
Saturated fats and trans fats are the ones everyone should try to cut down. They are the fats associated with the highest risks to health.

Saturated fat is found in animal fats – lard, butter, suet, meats (including poultry skin), dairy products, eggs, and in coconut, palm and palm-kernel oils. They're also often used in processed food. You should reduce the quantity of saturated fat in your diet; it has been clearly shown to raise blood cholesterol levels significantly.

Trans fats or hydrogenated fats are the very worst. They are vegetable fats treated to make them solid at room temperature and they lurk in surprising places, so check labels and avoid products that include trans fats, hydrogenated or partially hydrogenated fats. They're found in biscuits and cakes; even ostensibly healthy products like cereal bars; some spreads and bread; and fast food is often cooked in hydrogenated fat. You should exclude them completely from your diet as they are definitely linked to high cholesterol levels and increased rates of heart disease and cancer.

must know

Condiments

Watch out for pickles and condiments if you are trying to cut down on salt – mustard, ketchup and soy sauce are usually high in salt, and so are stock cubes. If you are used to eating a lot of salt, cut down gradually and you'll find the change easier to accept.

Cholesterol

Cholesterol can be confusing. It is a type of fat found in the blood, and having high levels can make you susceptible to all sorts of problems, especially heart disease. Some blood cholesterol isn't harmful: this is HDL or 'good' cholesterol. The other kind, LDL or 'bad' cholesterol, is the one to really watch out for: it causes the formation of fatty deposits which clog arteries and lead to an increased risk of heart attacks and stroke.

Saturated fats raise both types of cholesterol, which is why you should cut down on those, and trans fats do the same. On the other hand, polyunsaturates appear to lower both kinds of cholesterol and monounsaturates are the best – they lower the bad, LDL cholesterol and are thought to actually increase the proportion of HDL cholesterol in the blood, which is a good thing.

Watching blood-sugar levels and keeping your insulin production steady can help here too; when insulin levels are high, the level of HDL cholesterol in the blood goes down, which you don't want.

must know

Snacking

Unplanned snacks can ruin your diet so keep healthy ones, like fresh fruit or low-fat natural yoghurt, readily available.

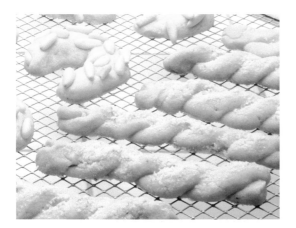

The trick with treats is to be able to stop. Restrict yourself to one and if you know you can't, then don't start.

Vitamins and minerals

Micronutrients (so called because we only need them in very small quantities) are just as important as carbs, proteins and fats. We all need a wide range of vitamins and minerals. Though we need to consider them, most of us will get what we require from our diet if we eat a wide range of healthy foods. Avoiding or reducing processed foods will help. Check the chart opposite and try to make sure that you are eating some food containing each vitamin or mineral on a regular basis. Some experts also suggest taking a daily multivitamin as an insurance policy.

Salt

Consuming too much salt is very common, but it's very bad too. It's associated with abnormally high blood pressure, and that increases the risk of developing a serious heart condition or having a stroke. The recommended total daily salt intake is 6g, just over a level teaspoon. Most people eat nearly double that, and most of the excess comes from processed food and ready meals. Just because something doesn't taste very salty doesn't mean there's no salt in it – many sweet biscuits contain some, for example. Here are a few easy-to-follow suggestions for cutting back your salt intake.

• Avoid manufactured foods wherever possible.

• Read food labels. Salt is shown as sodium and you have to multiply the weight by 2.5 to get the amount of salt. Look for less than 0.1 g of sodium per portion.

• Cut down on all fatty and salty foods – most are high in calories too, so there's a double benefit in cutting down. Smoked and cured foods like bacon, sausages and smoked fish are often very high in salt; their fresh equivalents have only a small amount.

• Rinse canned food and don't buy food canned in brine unless the only alternative is oil.

• Reduce the quantity of salt you use in cooking and don't add salt at the table.

Vitamins and minerals

Vitamin A Eggs, butter, fish oils, dark green and yellow fruits and vegetables, liver.
Essential for: strong bones, good eyesight, healthy skin, healing.

Vitamin B1 (Thiamine) Plant and animal foods, especially wholegrain products, brown rice, seafood and beans.
Essential for: growth, nerve function, conversion of blood sugar into energy.

Vitamin B2 (Riboflavin) Milk and dairy produce, green leafy vegetables, liver, kidneys, yeast.
Essential for: cell growth and reproduction, energy production.

Vitamin B3 (Niacin) Meats, fish and poultry, whole grains, peanuts and avocados.
Essential for: digestion, energy, the nervous system.

Vitamin B5 (Pantothenic acid) Organ meats, fish, eggs, chicken, nuts and wholegrain cereals.
Essential for: strengthening immunity and fighting infections, healing wounds.

Vitamin B6 (Pyridoxine) Meat, eggs, wholegrains, yeast, cabbage, melon, molasses.
Essential for: the production of new cells, a healthy immune system, production of antibodies and white blood cells.

Vitamin B12 (Cobalamin) Fish, dairy produce, beef, pork, lamb, organ meats, eggs and milk; vegans need to take supplements.
Essential for: energy and concentration, production of red blood cells, growth in children.

Vitamin C Fresh fruit and vegetables, potatoes, leafy herbs and berries.
Essential for: healthy skin, bones, muscles, healing, eyesight and protection from viruses.

Vitamin D Milk and dairy produce, eggs, fatty fish.
Essential for: healthy teeth and bones, vital for growth.

Vitamin E Nuts, seeds, eggs, milk, wholegrains, leafy vegetables, avocados and soya.
Essential for: absorption of iron and essential fatty acids, slowing the ageing process, increasing fertility.

Vitamin K Green vegetables, milk and dairy produce, apricots, wholegrains, cod liver oil.
Essential for: blood clotting.

Calcium Dairy produce, leafy green vegetables, salmon, nuts, root vegetables, tofu.
Essential for: strong bones and teeth, hormones and muscles, blood clotting and the regulation of blood pressure.

Iron Liver, kidney, cocoa powder, dark chocolate, shellfish, pulses, dark green vegetables, egg yolks, red meat, beans, molasses.
Essential for: supply of oxygen to the cells and a healthy immune system.

Magnesium Brown rice, soya beans, nuts, whole grains, bitter chocolate, legumes.
Essential for: transmission of nerve impulses, development of bones, growth and repair of cells.

Potassium Avocados, leafy green vegetables, bananas, fruit and vegetable juices, potatoes and nuts.
Essential for: maintaining water balance, nerve and muscle function.

Selenium Brazil nuts, fish, whole grains, garlic, mushrooms, cruciferous vegetables.
Essential for: normal cell growth, regulation of hormones, protection against cancer and immunity against infections like colds and flu.

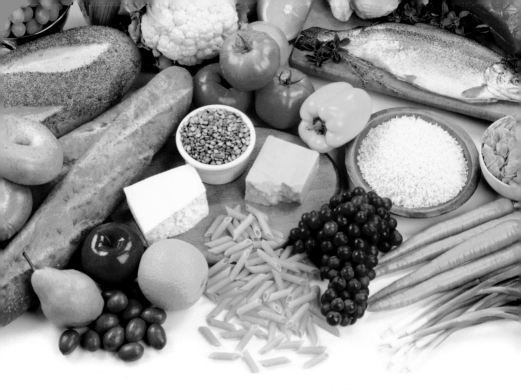

Eat a balanced range of foods for the good of your health as well as your diet.

must know

Fizzy pop

Watch sugary drinks, especially for children and teenagers. Those who drink just a can a day are significantly heavier than those who don't. Swap to low-calorie versions at the very least, or substitute with fresh juices and water.

• Use more herbs and spices instead.

• Check your breakfast cereal and if necessary swap to one lower in salt; many are quite high.

• Finally, it's possible to buy salt substitutes but they contain potassium, which should be avoided by anyone with kidney problems.

Sugar and sweeteners

Limit your intake of sugar as much as you can. It provides little in nutritional terms, is high in calories and has such an immediate effect on blood-sugar levels that it's at the top of many GI/GL scales and is used as the food that others are measured against. Unfortunately it also tastes really good. Try and wean yourself off sugar as much as you can as it's quite clear that eating too much of it is linked to overweight and obesity. Again, moderating the amount of processed food and ready meals should automatically reduce sugar levels, because many are very high in it. It is important that you read labels, but you should be aware of the fact that sugar can be described in many ways, such as dextrose, maltose, malto-dextrin, glucose syrup (anything described as a syrup is high in sugar), invert sugar and levulose. There are others, too.

Many people are reluctant to use artificial sweeteners, because research into their safety often produces contradictory results so it's difficult to assess how safe they actually are. If you really want the sugary taste you may prefer to switch to fructose, fruit sugar. It has the same calories as ordinary sugar, but it's much sweeter so you don't need as much. It's also becoming easy to find; health-food shops usually stock it, and so do some supermarkets now.

Drink

Somehow we feel as though drinking shouldn't really involve calories – unfortunately it does, and often lots of them. And it's not just alcohol, either. There's always a tendency to forget the cups of tea and coffee with milk and maybe sugar, and yet those can add significantly to your daily calorie count. Remember to think about what you're drinking as well as what you're eating.

First, it's crucial to keep your liquid intake up. Every part of the body requires water; every single cell needs it in order to function. The general recommen-dation is to drink at least six to eight glasses of still water every day. That's just plain water, though you could count herb tea. Flavoured water is often sugary, as are soft drinks, and tea and coffee are generally excluded because of the caffeine they contain.

must know

Labels

Watch some of the quick descriptions on labels. There are no legal definitions of 'low', 'reduced' or 'high', so treat labels that say 'low fat' and 'reduced sugar' with caution. A product cannot be described as 'reduced calorie' unless it is much lower-calorie than the normal version, but be careful. Check out the detailed information panels and compare different products' counts per 100g, not per portion.

You need more liquid when the weather is hot or in any circumstances where you perspire a lot, such as during exercise. Keep a bottle of water with you during the day. You can also sip from it when you get the urge to snack – there's some evidence that people can confuse the feeling of thirst for one of hunger, so not only will this keep you hydrated, it will also help you to cut down on calories.

Water is best. Cold soft drinks can be very harmful on a diet because many are stuffed with sugar. It really is best to cut right down on these. One recent piece of research bears this out: teenagers who have a can of sugary drink every day are likely to be nearly 6.5kg – nearly a whole stone – heavier after a year than those who drink low-calorie versions. This warning doesn't just apply to adolescents but to adults as well.

Watch how much milk you add to tea and coffee, or take tea with lemon rather than milk. Lemon is particularly good with more delicate teas like Earl Grey. You could check out green teas, much praised for their antioxidant qualities, as they don't need milk, and there are many delicious flavours of herbal teas. Try to get used to the taste of black coffee – it's much easier to appreciate the taste of different coffees without milk, and they can be very different, so experiment and find ones you like. The other thing about coffee, particularly, is caffeine. Some dietitians specifically recommend decaffeinated coffee and tea because increased caffeine leads to increased insulin production. If you want to cut down, it may be best to do it gradually. Try using a smaller cup at first.

Alcohol can be a minefield for any dieter. Some diets suggest you abandon the idea of drinking alcohol when you're dieting, but if that would be too painful, you can think about cutting it down. After all, alcohol provides no nutritional benefits (though some health benefits have been attributed to red wine), can be high in calories – and several drinks can make you forget about dieting altogether. There's no doubt that cutting it out

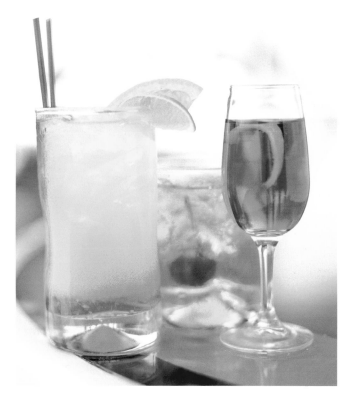

Give dieters and non-drinkers a treat with different kinds of delicious fruit juice cocktails.

completely will help your weight loss. However, if that would be a sacrifice too far, here's some advice on how to stop it wrecking your low-calorie diet.

It's easy to forget to tot up the calories for any alcohol you drink over the course of an evening, so watch it and keep tabs. Always use low-calorie mixers when they're available. Measures of spirits are another problem. If you are ordering in most pubs and clubs you can be sure how much spirit you'll get in your glass – a standard single or double measure. At home, however, it's all too easy to slosh it in, so invest in an accurate drinks measure and count calories accordingly. And be wary of drinks poured by someone else, too – it's probably best to stick to a small glass of wine in this case.

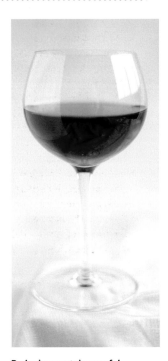

Red wine contains useful antioxidants - but go easy.

Moderation is the best, so try and think of alcohol as a treat when you're trying to lose weight. One of the best things you can do is to make sure you only drink when you are eating. Alcohol is absorbed through the stomach wall so it enters the blood-stream quickly, ultimately resulting in increased insulin production and consequent feelings of hunger, and this can happen quickly – everyone knows how easy it is to get drunk on an empty stomach. Eating something relatively substantial, either beforehand or at the same time, will slow the process down.

Now for what to drink. Beer is worth avoiding, as it can be very high in calories. Go for dry wines, preferably red because of the health benefits, and avoid sweeter wine, beer, lager and particularly stout. Spirits can be problematic if you don't monitor the quantity, and the same is true of liqueurs, some of which are shockingly sweet. They can, however, be very useful in desserts and puddings, especially as a substitute for fruit syrups in fresh fruit salad. Measuring is the important thing.

And finally...

Sometimes eating healthily can seem very confusing. It doesn't have to be. Here's a quick round-up of the best advice:
• If something contains ingredients you don't recognize or can't even pronounce, don't buy it.
• Eat your five portions of fruit and veg a day; try to eat more. Don't drown your fruit and veg with high-calorie sauces containing butter or cream.
• Avoid refined grains; automatically go for whole-grain products.

• Avoid processed foods and ready meals. The saying goes that if you can pick it, dig it or kill it, then it's probably healthy for you.
• Avoid trans fats completely, saturated fats as much as is humanly possible, and watch out for full-fat dairy products because they are high in saturates (and calories).
• Cut right down on salt and sugar.
• Include as wide a range of foods as possible in your diet – with the exception of the foods you are advised to avoid, of course.
• Drink plenty of fluids and be sensible about alcohol.
• Be good 80 per cent of the time. It's likely to be good enough.

Knowing what to eat, and related details like the effect it will have on your body, is all very well – but you need to know how to put your knowledge into practice when you are watching the calories. Fortunately there is loads of practical information that you can use to make calorie counting as painless as possible... and it's in the next chapter, so read on.

want to know more?

• In chapter 8 you'll find calorie counts for common foods. For a fuller, handbag-sized listing of calories, get the *Collins Gem Calorie Counter*.

websites

• You'll find plenty of nutritional information on the Web. Check out www.eatwell.gov.uk and www.bbc.co.uk/health/healthy_living/nutrition – they are both packed with advice.
• www.5aday.nhs.uk has information about the government's fruit and veg campaign.
• www.vegsoc.org/info/foodfacts.html has advice on healthy eating for vegetarians.
• See also the box on page 74 for a list of useful nutrition websites.

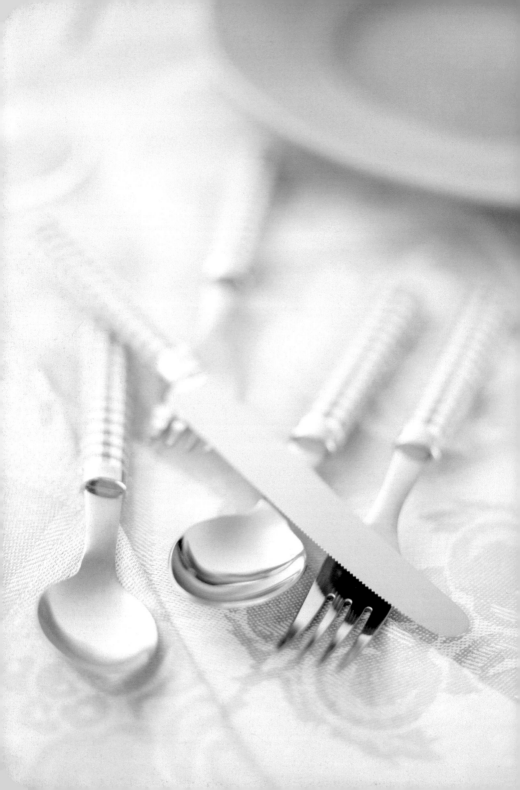

5 Calorie counting in practice

When you're calorie counting, you don't need to know what you're going to be doing two weeks on Thursday, as you do with some diets. You can be as creative as you want, but you do have to be a little disciplined about it. This is the crucial part: how to combine the freedom and flexibility that calorie counting gives you with enough structure to make it work, but not so much that it fails.

Calorie counting in practice

There are lots of ways to make calorie counting easier. Let's look at the whole process from actually starting your diet through to maintaining your brand new weight.

Knowledge is power

We saw how to work out a realistic target in chapter 2. Now's the time to revisit that, but it helps if you have some idea of where potential problems might lie before you start. The very first step, before you count a single calorie, is to keep a basic food diary. It doesn't have to be for days or weeks, just for two typical days, one at the weekend and one during the week.

You'll need to do a bit of weighing and measuring. For everything you eat or drink, except water, note:
• the time
• what it was, and be as specific as possible - '100g cornflakes with 50ml whole milk', for example, not just 'bowl of cereal'
• why you ate it - this may sound obvious but can be very helpful, and it can cover things like 'bored', 'starving' and 'needing chocolate on way home'
• how hungry you actually were; grade it, if you wish, on a scale of 1–10.

Now you need to get hold of a calorie counter. There are various ones about, generally all reasonably priced, and you'll probably find you need a couple to cover everything. The *Collins Gem Calorie Counter* has other nutritional information in it as well, which can be useful, and there are values for basic foods in the listings section of this book. You'll probably find you end up using the nutritional info' on food packaging sometimes, too. This will all become automatic, second nature, so don't let yourself be distracted by it at this stage. Freedom is worth it!

Sit down with your food diary and work out your calories for the two days; a small calculator will probably be useful. There are bound to be some vague areas – 'milky coffee' for example – but despite that you'll probably be surprised by the total. Most of us take in far more energy than we use, so remind yourself of how much you are likely to be using by revisiting the rough assessment you made on pages 31-3. If you are eating more than your body is using, you will be putting weight on because of it.

Check the reasons why you ate certain foods. Remarks like 'starving to death' in mid-afternoon mean that you either didn't have enough lunch,

on pages 31-3.

must know

Muesli

Muesli 'weighs very heavy' – the portion you might want to eat may well blow your calorie count for the day. Think about adding some fresh fruit to a smaller quantity. Nectarines are ideal and a bit different, and you'll eat fewer calories than you would if you added more muesli.

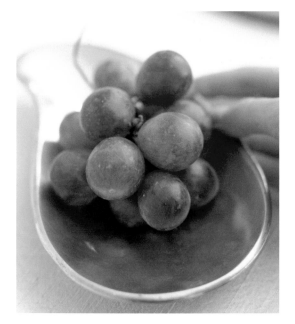

Black grapes are delicious frozen. Wash them, shake them dry and pop small bunches in the freezer.

Doctors sometimes use calipers to assess body fat - a more technical version of the informal 'pinch an inch' test.

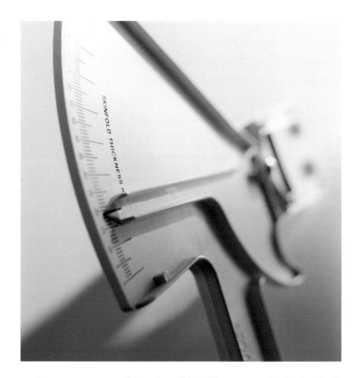

or that you ate something that didn't fill you up - foods that had a swift effect on your blood sugar. Notes like 'feeling stressed' or 'craving chocolate' are useful indicators of your flash points. It's important to remind yourself that crisps don't really help to reduce stress levels so try and address the real problem. Successful dieters often report that their diet has changed more than just their shape and health: it's empowering in other ways too. Your basic food diary is useful for highlighting bad habits, like the chocolate craving or late-afternoon crisp urges. Once you know your danger points you can work round them, so make a mental note of any you've developed.

Starting out

Weigh yourself first thing in the morning, after you go to the loo and before you have breakfast. Make a mental note of what you're wearing – pyjamas or preferably nothing. Have bare feet and make sure the scales are level on hard flooring. When you weigh yourself in future, wear the same clothes (or lack of them) and have the scales in the same place. Scales used by many different people, like those in a fitness centre, or by children playing on them, or very heavy men bouncing on and off, may well not be accurate.

You might want to make a note of your measurements at this time too: remember that muscle weighs more than fat, and you may well want to have more than one way of assessing change as you trim up. Measure your waist, hips, chest, thighs and upper arms and note down the figures.

Chapter 2 looked at how to give yourself a reasonable target, and at how much to eat to get there. Now's the time to put this information into practice, so let's recap.

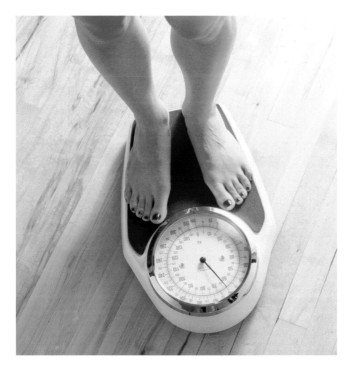

Invest in the best scales you can afford, and always use the same ones.

must know

Measuring milk

Pour some milk into a measuring jug and only use that for your drinks during the day. At night you can measure how much is left. This will give you a basic idea of how much you need to allow for in your daily calorie total, but watch out for days when you drink an abnormally large number of cups of milky tea. Guesswork could make a significant difference, especially if you're still using full-cream milk.

If you're a woman:
• with less than 6.5kg to lose – 1250 calories per day
• with 6.5–19kg to lose – 1500 calories per day
• with over 19kg to lose – 1750 calories per day

If you're a man:
• with less than 6.5kg to lose – 1500 calories per day
• with 6.5–19kg to lose – 1750 calories per day
• with over 19kg to lose – 2000 calories per day

On pages 60-1 two changes were described that can make a difference without counting a single calorie – cutting down on junk food (fast food or unhealthy snacks) and any processed food and ready meals. There are some tips coming up which will help you to take control of your consumption of convenience foods. Now for the nitty-gritty.

Counting your calories

You need to think about how to divide your calories throughout the day. From your food diary you'll know, for example, if you really need a little snack in mid-evening, so you can build that in. Be flexible, though: as your diet becomes healthier and more satisfying you may find that your appetite changes.

There's a simple rule here which will make your dieting life easier – always have breakfast, lunch and dinner. Never, ever, starve yourself or skip meals as it will only bring on bingeing and the end of your dieting resolve. Make your diet work for you; make it as easy as possible for you to succeed.

As far as breakfast is concerned, many studies have demonstrated the importance of this meal in enabling and sustaining weight loss, so make it a priority not to skip it.

Here are a couple of breakdowns; yours doesn't have to look like either of them, of course. Don't forget to allow for milk in drinks – once you see it in black and white you may decide to go for black coffee and tea with lemon!

	1250 calories	1500 calories
Breakfast	250	300
Morning snack	100	none
Lunch	350	400
Afternoon snack	100	100
Dinner	350	500
Evening snack	none	100
Milk all day	100	100

You'll find some meal and snack suggestions in chapter 6, and calorie-counted recipes in chapter 7.

At some point every calorie-counting dieter falls into the trap of running out of calories part way through the day. If this happens to you – make sure

must know

Cheese

Cheese is easy to nibble, easy to prepare and could make an ideal snack, but it is loaded with calories. Try low-fat cheeses, or go for smaller quantities of stronger-tasting ones. But whatever you do, monitor your cheese intake carefully.

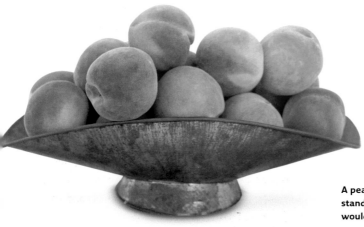

A peach is 50 calories while a standard-size chocolate bar would be about 300.

it isn't often – don't starve yourself. Have something healthy to tide you over, maybe an apple, a low-fat yoghurt or a slice of wholemeal toast. Don't punish yourself as it won't work, but try to keep your blood-sugar level as steady as possible without eating lots.

The best way of keeping tabs on what you're doing is planning. Yes, calorie counting does give you freedom, but it also demands that you take control. Think a little (but don't obsess) about what you are going to eat a day beforehand. Sort out a packed lunch if you need to, and just consider how you're going to use your calories. On the day itself – and this is crucial, particularly at the start – record them.

Keeping a record

The importance of keeping a record of what you eat while you're actively counting calories can't be overstressed. If it sounds tedious, don't worry – it soon becomes marginal, a habit. It's also extremely useful for helping you to become calorie-aware, almost without realizing it. As things become second nature you might feel you can give up record-keeping, but monitor your weight loss carefully if you do and return to recording if it speeds up too much, slows down or stalls.

Make a blank table on a sheet of A4 paper. It should be divided into seven horizontal rows, one for each day of the week and needs five vertical columns, a thin one at each end and three thicker ones in the middle. Photocopy it and keep your original safe. The first column is where you write the day, and the last one is where you enter the total calories. In between write what you're eating and its calorie value.

Now there is a syndrome called dietary amnesia. You can genuinely forget eating the odd biscuit, so be sure to record everything as soon after you eat it as possible. One of the most frequently forgotten things is also one of the most calorific – alcohol. Make notes at the time if necessary and fill in your main record later, but don't rely on your memory. If you stopped record keeping and have put weight on, this might be the problem; the things you don't remember could be undermining your diet. And, whatever else you do with your record, be honest and as accurate as possible. There are some shortcut tips coming up.

If you wish, you can record your weight at the start of each week but you don't have to judge weight loss by the scales. In fact some people find it a positive hindrance – if the scales show a loss, they feel they can let themselves go, and if they show a gain they get depressed and stop dieting. If that sounds like you, then judge your weight loss by the fit of your clothes instead. If you do opt for using scales then don't weigh yourself more than once a week and accept that there might be some fluctuations that are nothing to do with your diet (most women find their weight varies with their menstrual cycle, for example). Look at trends over three or four weeks instead.

Once you start monitoring what you are eating, you can easily check the balance of your diet on your record and adjust it if necessary. Are you getting at least five portions of fruit and veg a day? Is there some healthy protein in there? Have sweets sneaked in?

If you find you're having problems, expand your record to be more of a food diary like the one you kept for a couple of days before starting. How was your mood when you ate that snack? Maybe there's something you need to resolve. And if you were roaring hungry by mid-morning and just had to have a king-size chocolate bar, then something evidently went adrift with your breakfast; try changing it.

Record-keeping shortcuts
The following tips should help you to keep a good record of what you eat. Come up with your own ideas, too – as time goes by you'll get to know the figures for your favourite foods and most

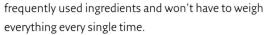

Raspberries

Raspberries have lots of fibre, plenty of vitamin C, small amounts of iron and B vitamins – and are low in calories. But don't spoil it by smothering them in lots of cream and sugar; if you let them warm rather than eating them straight from the fridge, you'll find the flavour really comes through without any extras.

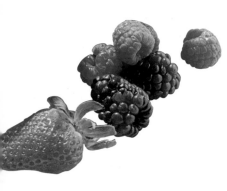

frequently used ingredients and won't have to weigh everything every single time.

• Don't get trapped into nitpicking: a tablespoon of skimmed milk is 4.8 calories, but round it up to 5. Whole milk is double the calories of skimmed.

• A teaspoon of olive oil (or any other oil, come to that) is between 40 and 45 calories

• A medium tangerine is 25 calories, a mandarin is 30, a medium orange is 56.

• A small apple is 50, an average pear 60.

• Watch dried fruit: each dried apricot is about 10–15 calories depending on size, but each date is approximately 30 and a dried fig 45. A level tablespoon of raisins or sultanas is 40.

• A medium plum is 36, a fresh apricot 16, and a medium peach 50.

• A small-to-medium onion, trimmed and peeled, is about 100g – 36 calories.

• An average tomato is 29 and a single cherry tomato would be only 5.

• A small egg is about 80, a medium egg 85, and a large one 100.

• Two back rashers of bacon, trimmed of excess fat, weigh about 75g (all rashers are different and thin ones would weigh much less); grilled and blotted of excess fat on kitchen paper the same two rashers weigh 40g – 86 calories.

• Some products come in convenient sizes. A Camembert, for example, is 250g and a whole one would be 725 calories. An eighth is easy to cut and comes in at a convenient snack level – 90 calories. A mini Babybel is 60.

• Heaped spoon measures make a huge difference. A heaped tablespoon of low-calorie mayo could be as much as 150 calories if you really went for it. A level one would be about 45. Ordinary mayo would be 105 for a level tablespoonful.

• A standard croissant is about 250 calories, a mini one 125, and a pain au chocolat could be about 275. The raisin equivalent can be as much as 380. Danish pastries are generally worse.

Then a few general points:

• Never forget to add whatever you use to cook food with. A raw, skinless chicken breast may be low-calorie, but cook it in two tablespoons of oil and you're adding more calories than the chicken itself (about 115 for the chicken, 270 for the oil).

• As a quick guide for meat, remember that the more fat it contains, the higher it will be in calories.

• Once again, there is a tendency to forget to add calories from drinks, so be aware of this and be careful. A pub measure (25ml) of a spirit – gin, whisky, rum, vodka – is 56 calories, and a 150ml glass of red wine is just over 100. You could follow a rough guide if you had to: a finger of spirit is about 25ml, but don't rely on this. When you're thinking about nibbles while you drink, a plain olive is 3 calories and a stuffed one 5; a single brazil nut is 25, the same as a single cashew. Over to you!

Shopping for food

There are some basic guidelines which can make shopping more diet-friendly. Some are obvious, some perhaps less so. Firstly, even the most virtuous of us would be tempted by unsuitable food if we went shopping when hungry, so remember the mantra: set yourself up to succeed and eat first. But the effects of being hungry when you shop don't

must know

Snack foods

Make sure any snacks you eat fit into your daily calorie allowance. Keep high-calorie snack food out of your kitchen as much as possible because if something is there you are more likely to be tempted...

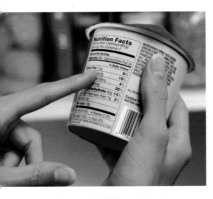

Check the full nutritional information panel on all packaged foods.

stop at the supermarket shelf; you're also much more likely to snack in the car or when you unpack at home. Make it easy for yourself – never, ever, go food shopping on an empty stomach. If you habitually weaken, then don't buy the things that tempt you.

Try to avoid impulse food shopping, which can make it easier to cave in. Make lists of what you need and don't allow yourself to buy non-essential extras. You can also stop yourself from impulse purchasing by reading labels: if you don't recognize an ingredient, have no idea what it is and can't even pronounce it, put the product back.

Labels are useful for dieters, but follow a few guidelines. Don't ever rely on the brief description flashed on the front of a product, but check out the full nutritional information too. Some cereal bars are labelled 'healthy' but still contain large amounts of sugar; 'active' yoghurt drinks often contain a surprising amount of sugar – about 13g per 100g for the plain ones. The flavoured ones are higher. When you're looking at the nutritional info' panels, check out the 'per 100g' figures, especially if you're comparing brands, as manufacturers' portions are arbitrary – some can be very small, so be aware of that too. A 'meal for two' may actually only be enough for one, but the calories per portion will be for half the total quantity. The 'per item' figures are useful when looking at things like biscuits, though, and can be pretty scary. Chocolate bars which are split into two or more bars may have a figure for one bar – but can you really stop at one? – so check those carefully as well.

If you are a butter user and don't fancy life without a substitute, change to a low-fat spread, but check

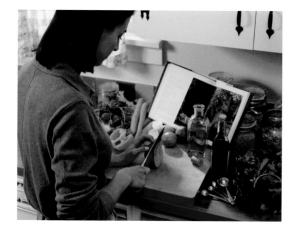

If you cook for yourself, using fresh ingredients, you'll be healthier – and more likely to succeed on your diet.

that it is high in the right sort of fats. Compare the nutritional information per 100g of product across different brands, and check out the olive oil spreads, too (see pages 74-6 for information on which fats to choose). When it comes to bread, help yourself by buying sliced loaves – you can freeze the slices in pairs. Though these can be toasted straight from the freezer, they are more difficult to snack on without thinking. It is also easier to judge portions if the bread is sliced.

Cooking

Cooking for yourself is one of the best ways to succeed and it's enjoyable – especially as most people who have a weight problem love their food. Try and make time for it, as it really is vital.

Boredom can undermine even the most determined, committed dieter. One of the clear ways to avoid this is to vary what you eat, and even better, to cook it yourself. Eat the same thing every day, or every few days, and the chances are that you'll fail. This especially applies to using ready meals and

must know

Cooking time

If you think you haven't got enough time to cook, do the telly test. How much time do you spend watching the television in a week? Allocate just half an hour a day of that time to spend in the kitchen.

processed foods, where manufacturers want to achieve uniformity – they need to know that one pack of lasagne is going to taste the same as the next. If you are more creative than that about what you eat, you are more likely to be successful at weight loss.

It is important not to feel isolated when you are dieting, so it is best to eat broadly the same things as anybody you may share your meal with; non-dieters can add extra accompaniments – rice, pasta, potatoes, whatever they wish. This also has the advantage of ensuring that you, the dieter, don't feel too tempted or ill-done-by. Nothing is more guaranteed to invite disaster than sitting at the table eating lettuce and feeling like a martyr when everyone else is chomping on chips. Cooking the same thing for everybody helps. You can get the whole family eating healthily, after all.

Again, simple things can make your life easier. First, however, get the measuring right. 'Slimmers' measuring scales are worth getting; they only weigh relatively small quantities but show these far more clearly than standard scales do, and they are usually fairly cheap. A set of measuring spoons is also useful as ordinary spoons can vary. The standard measures are 15ml for a tablespoon and 5ml for a teaspoon. A rounded spoonful of something will contain many more calories, so assume that a level spoonful is intended, unless a recipe says otherwise.

Always use non-stick pans. You need very little oil or fat when cooking in them – you could even experiment with an oil spray – and can usually cut the quantities given in any 'non-dieting' recipe without seriously affecting the taste. Some food, like bacon, will cook successfully in a non-stick pan without needing any extra fat at all, and you can even fry an egg in the same pan.

Many recipes in books and magazines give the calorie values, but make sure that you know whether the values are per portion – and if so, check how many people each dish is supposed to serve – or per dish. Follow the quantities given unless you do

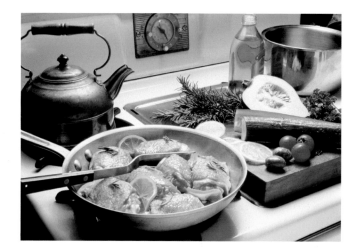

Chicken is good, but don't forget to remove the skin when you're dieting. It reduces both the calories and the amount of saturated fat.

something simple like halve them to serve two instead of four, but be careful to get the sums right if you do. If you change the quantity, cooking times may be affected so checking that things are properly cooked is even more important than usual.

Adapting recipes from non-dieting cookery books is easy; it may also help on the time front as most recipes these days need nothing more than a bit of planning and relatively little time when you're actually cooking. With ordinary recipes, examine the ingredients and decide what you should cut. Fats are often particularly high in calories – ask yourself if a particular recipe really needs six tablespoons of olive oil and if it does seem to, then move on to something else.

Most of the time quantities of fatty ingredients can be hacked back savagely without any unpleasant effects on the final taste. Soup is easy to adapt, especially if you avoid recipes containing lots of potato and cream. Most soup is traditionally made by initially frying some of the ingredients, often in a lot of oil or butter. This oil can be reduced to the minimum if you use a non-stick pan, or it can even be omitted altogether; just add the ingredients to good stock. If you do adapt any recipes you will need to get out your calculator, though, to work out the calories for yourself. Changing ingredients may also affect cooking times. Don't automatically cut, though.

Extra portions can be frozen in some cases; soups and casseroles freeze particularly well. Be wary of freezing foods that may get overcooked when you reheat them – spinach is a good example as it can get unpalatably slimy. Frozen dishes make useful home-made ready meals, a great dieting shortcut which will also help you to avoid bought ready meals and processed food. Write on the freezer container what the dish is and how many calories it contains, and put the date on as well. Spicy dishes become spicier with freezing, so you may want to use those fairly quickly.

There are a few more potential pitfalls to consider. Weigh high-calorie ingredients like rice and pasta carefully as a small error could mean a lot of extra calories. With pasta – and this applies to eating out as well – choose vegetable sauces and avoid those with lots of cream, butter or cheese; don't sprinkle tons of Parmesan on the top, either. Check out wholemeal pastas, as they are lower in calories and will fill you up more effectively. You also need to be very careful about cheese generally, because it is so high in calories and mismeasuring is easy.

Always remove chicken skin as not only does it reduce the calorie count, it also significantly reduces the amount of saturated fat. Cut visible fat off other meats and if you usually buy mince, make sure you select very lean kinds and cook off the fat before using it in a recipe. Beef and lamb mince are similar in nutritional terms, but lamb mince is a more authentic choice when you are making Middle-Eastern or Indian dishes – check it out.

How to eat

Some diet books are full of recommendations about how you should eat. There are tips about slowing down and valuing your food more: for example, 'put your cutlery down between each mouthful' and 'concentrate on the taste of every mouthful'; these are supposed to make it easier to diet, but they may not work for everyone – however, be aware that tips like this might just help.

In general, if you are paying more attention to a healthy diet, you are already appreciating your food more. It is worth making sure that you eat without distractions like watching television at the same time – make a meal a bit more special than that. An apparently daft tip that can work is never eating when you're standing up. Sounds simple, but it's effective – you cut down on things like tasting when you're cooking, snacking on leftovers as you clear up, and absent-mindedly polishing off a chocolate bar at the bus stop.

Potential problems

It's impossible to stick to a regime all the time, so remember that and don't blame yourself unnecessarily if you do slip a little. Here's some guidance on common problem areas and difficulties.

Bad habits

Your food diary will have helped you to pinpoint these, but you probably know about them anyway. Break them. You can do it – it takes three weeks, they say, to actually break the habit and another three to stop thinking about the fact that you've broken it and harking after it. Here's an example. If your first action

Sit at the table to eat your meal rather than balancing it on your lap in front of the TV, where you may not even notice what you're eating.

must knows

Olives

Olives are a much better nibble than peanuts. Buy plain ones in brine; rinse them well, add some fresh herbs and a brief drizzle of olive oil, and let them sit for a few minutes to absorb the flavours.

on coming home from work is to have a large glass of wine and some crisps, then break the routine by doing something else, like going and changing out of your work clothes. Then work out when you are on automatic snacking pilot – those moments when you find yourself having a quick biscuit 'just because'. Habits like those could be ruining your diet, so recognize and change them.

Cravings, bingeing and boredom (again)

Cravings can be avoided by sticking to a pattern of regular meals and a couple of snacks a day as they are most likely to strike when you've allowed yourself to get too hungry – and then they are very difficult to resist. The most important thing to do is consider it seriously, as trying to avoid thinking about 'the elephant in the room' doesn't work. Do you really want to put your diet in jeopardy for that mega bag of tortilla chips? Another strong-tasting savoury snack could stop something like that one in its tracks – try a little anchovy paste on an oatcake, for example. It's always worth trying to stop yourself because many cravings can lead to … bingeing.

Anybody who diets will binge at some point. Learn to recognize the signs of a binge developing; it's most likely to happen when you're bored, depressed, tired, irritable or frustrated. Physical activity is a great way to prevent a binge, and so is breaking a pattern by doing something like leaving the house for a few minutes. If you don't manage to avoid it, then don't try and compensate by eating very little the following day as you'll just feel outrageously hungry, which will weaken your resolve, and then you'll be craving that little something. If your diet

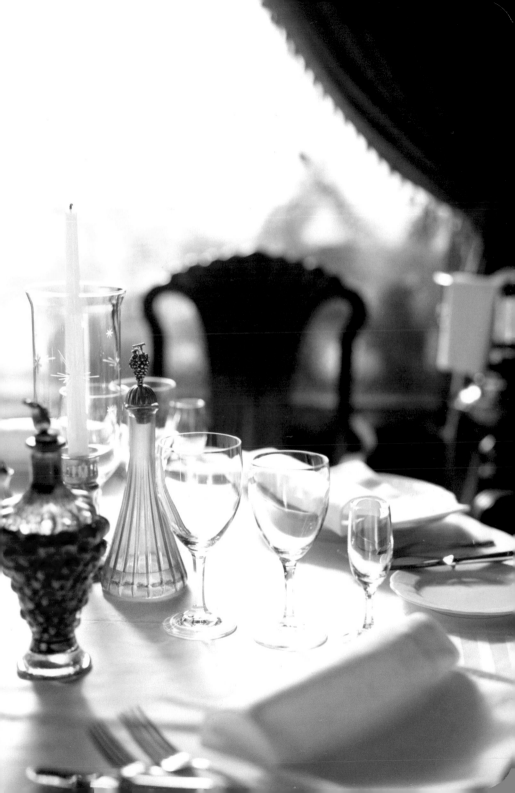

Barbecue food can be fine for your diet, but watch out for lavish salad dressings and all those burger buns and sauces.

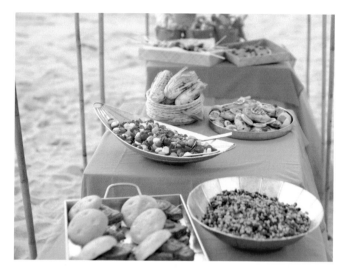

goes astray for one day, don't abandon it. Get back on it the next day; you might be tempted to cut back on the calories to compensate, but don't do that too much. It's more important to think about whether there was a real trigger. Are you getting too hungry? If so, look at the carb content of your diet and make sure you are eating enough whole grains and unrefined carbs.

If you find binges becoming a real problem, you might want to think about getting some external help and learning more about eating disorders (see box on page 108); sometimes the line can be a thin one.

Boredom, as mentioned earlier, is the other major problem, but this is boredom in general, not just boredom with the food you're eating. Lots of people eat if they get bored, so if you find yourself absent-mindedly drifting towards the fridge or the biscuit tin, do something else. Go for a quick walk, leave the room, whatever works for you – it doesn't matter what you do so long as you distract yourself. Make a cup of tea. Do that little job you've been meaning to do all day. The same applies at work; it's very easy to be drawn to a vending machine without really thinking about what you are doing.

Plateauing

Most successful dieters have experienced this effect. You've been losing weight steadily and then you seem to stick and nothing works. You can cut your intake, push your exercise up, but still nothing shifts. Plateaus will be more of a problem if you've dieted a lot in the past. They are caused by your body trying to protect itself from potential disaster, trying to conserve as much energy as possible since it thinks it's in a survival situation. They are also caused by losing too much weight too quickly, for exactly the same reasons.

It may be that you are trying to get down to too low a weight, so check your aims again. Then, most importantly, stop panicking. Stop cutting calories aggressively, stop exercising like a mad thing – give yourself a break and relax. You need to get back in sympathy with your body and not push it too far, too fast. Some serious studies have shown that a three-month break from a diet can be very effective, so try not to put any weight back on and have a breather.

Quitting

If you feel like giving up, think seriously about why – it might be just an minor excuse, not something fundamentally serious. Everyone who has dieted has experienced the 'what's the point?' moment, often after a binge. Remember why you wanted to lose weight in the first place and if you made a list, re-read it. Think about the weight you've already lost – do you really want to put that back on? And then some time in the future try to lose it again, with all the problems that can bring? Losing weight is a real achievement, so don't waste it.

Then reward yourself. It does sound demented, but if you're going to stick with your diet, pat yourself on the back. Do something you'd really enjoy, something indulgent. You could have a manicure, or a sauna and massage, or spend ages choosing a luxurious new body lotion (don't even think about

must know

Eating disorders

If you think you may have a problem that's getting a bit much for you, check out www.eatingproblems .org and www.edauk .com, the website of the Eating Disorders Association. You'll find their address and telephone number on page 189.

rewarding yourself with food; you may have done that in the past, but that was then, not now). Marking dieting milestones also helps you to get used to accepting your new body.

Hiccups – holidays and the like

Every diet is punctuated by high days and holidays, and even eating out and parties, which can pose problems. But nothing is insurmountable; above all, don't use these as an excuse for stopping your diet.

Birthdays and holidays can all be problematic, but allow yourself a day off for your birthday, a couple of days off over Christmas and perhaps another one at Easter. It won't do too much damage unless you go completely mad – but don't eat up the leftovers for days and days; no little snacks of Christmas cake for weeks afterwards. Go back on your diet instead, having really enjoyed your time out. Don't try and diet when people all around you are stuffing their faces: remember – make it easy for yourself.

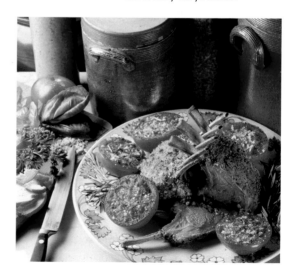

Choose wisely when you're on holiday, but don't let your diet dominate your time off.

When it comes to longer breaks, stop counting but be sensible. You don't need to quiz the taverna owner about what's gone into your meal, but you know enough to choose sensibly, and remember that it's easier if you don't drink until you've got something else in your stomach first. Steer clear of obviously high-calorie foods except as treats but do enjoy yourself all the same. Get back on your diet when you return. There are loads more eating out tips on pages 110-11.

Parties

Parties, whether on holiday or just because, may be difficult. If you don't want to give yourself time out from your diet, then follow these simple rules.

• Only drink alcohol if you're eating something, and limit yourself to a single glass if you can – top up with water thereafter.

• Never stand close to any food; this reduces the chance of idle nibbling while you chat.

• If you can't get out of nibbles, go for olives (if they're there) rather than bits of cheese, sausages or crisps. Otherwise there may be raw vegetables to use in dips – check those out.

• If you have a decent meal before you leave for the party, resisting food and excess alcohol when you're actually there will be a lot easier.

• Finally, have a dance. It's fun, good exercise and you can't eat or drink while you're doing it!

Eating out

If you're eating in a restaurant, sensible choices are necessary whatever the cuisine involved, but it's usually relatively easy. Whatever you do, don't try

must know

Party food

This can be a minefield. Anything involving pastry is out – a small pork pie can have nearly 400 calories, so even a slice is risky. Mini tartlets may be 70 calories or so each, and a small vol-au-vent might well be between 75 and 120 calories. Tiny sausage rolls are about 130, and they're very moreish. Don't forget the crisps – 25g of these is about the same as the sausage roll.

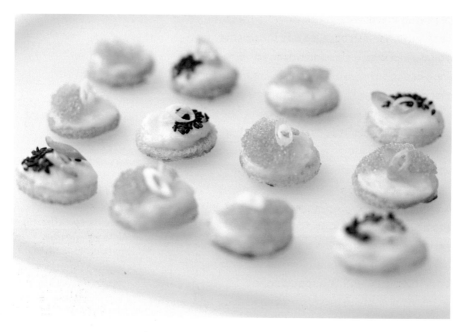

Avoid canapés made with bread, as the bread is often fried.

and guess calories; give yourself a break from counting. You can help by taking the edge off your appetite with an apple before you leave the house, which will make it easier to decline the offer of bread when you arrive. Have some water while you're looking at the menu, order wine by the glass, and never order pudding at the start.

Ask the waiter questions about cooking methods (if you're embarrassed, you could explain that you have a health problem and have to watch what you eat, particularly fat and/or sugar); most waiters will be happy to explain. You can ask for boiled new potatoes instead of chips, or boiled rice instead of fried. Ask for sauces to be served on the side or not at all, and request that your vegetables aren't served in butter, if it's that sort of restaurant.

Go for grilled meat or fish, look out for whole grains rather than refined carbs if at all possible; if not, keep your consumption of them to a minimum. Watch for the use of ghee (clarified butter) in Indian restaurants and go for tandoori dishes instead, but avoid any with thick sauces. That point is a good guide for Chinese food too – steamed dishes are the best option here – and is equally valid for French and Italian restaurants.

A few other points: firstly, never order avocado. Not only is it very high in calories itself – a half can be as much as 240 calories – it is also likely to come with a high-calorie dressing. Melon is delicious, and it makes a good dessert as well.

Salads can seem like a diet-friendly shortcut, but you never know exactly what's been added, so ask. Dressings, for instance, can add a lot of calories, so you should try to get oil and vinegar brought to the table separately. When it comes to menus and salad bars, watch out for and avoid anything obviously containing mayo, rice, pasta or lots of oil.

There's only one thing to do with pastry, whatever kind of restaurant you're in, from Greek to French to takeaways: avoid it. Pastry is very high in calories and fat, and usually it's the wrong kind of fat.

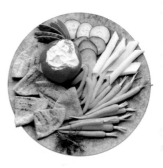

Crudités are an excellent choice when eating out, but fill up on the vegetables, not the dip!

Be careful that you're not just eating dessert because you're in the habit of doing so, and don't automatically have one – if you feel comfortably satisfied after your main course, stop. You may be able to have fresh fruit, though be careful of fruit salads which might be served in syrup. Meringues can be surprisingly low in calories because they are fatless, even though they are mostly sugar; the problem, though, is the thick cream which often accompanies them. Use your common sense; sorbets and water ices are generally an excellent option while fritters are not.

Finally, cheese and biscuits are often seen as a good dieting alternative to dessert, but cheese can ratchet up the calories alarmingly. Stilton is often included on a cheese platter in restaurants, and it is particularly high-calorie. Brie and Camembert are better options, but the best choice of all would be to go for fresh fruit instead, or just have coffee.

Maintaining your weight

At last – you got there and you got there gently. That should make sticking to your new weight easier. Now what?

Build up calories very gradually. You don't want to lose more – you really don't – but you don't want to put it on, either, and just after you get to target is a danger time. Remember that the way you used to eat is what made you overweight in the first place, so you're not going back to it.

Initially, allow yourself to eat about an extra 200 calories a day and see how it goes. Carry on weighing yourself once a week, if that's what you're happy with, and make sure that you get back in control if you slip. Do bear in mind that your weight will naturally fluctuate a little, but if you increase by

A few grilled prawns on top of a salad can make it look magnificent.

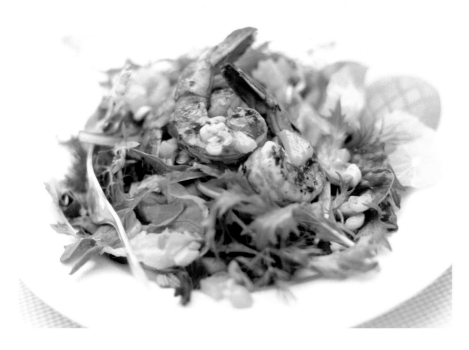

2kg or more, or if you find you're straining the seams of a garment which fitted easily when you were at your target, get back on the diet. Just spend a few days at it, as that should be enough.

If you stick with the healthy eating guidelines you've been following and watch any tendencies to slither out of them, keeping your weight steady should be possible.

Don't forget your exercise as this is the point at which the benefits really begin to show themselves, where the difference between non-exercisers and those who are more active is really clear. You are much, much more likely to keep to your new weight if you keep up your exercise routine.

Basically, monitor what you weigh but don't obsess about it, keep the faith on diet and exercise, make amendments if you need to – and congratulations!

want to know more?

• *Collins Gem Calorie Counter* lists not just calories, but other nutritional information as well – very useful when you're trying to eat healthily.
• For help when you've got to target, try www.bbc.co.uk/health/healthy_living/your_weight/reaching_maintaining.shtml.
• Don't forget about the role of exercise in keeping your weight down; re-read chapter 4.

websites
• www.caloriecounting.co.uk
• www.bupa.co.uk/health_information/asp/healthyliving/lifestyle/diet
• www.netdoctor.co.uk/health_advice/facts/loseweight.htm

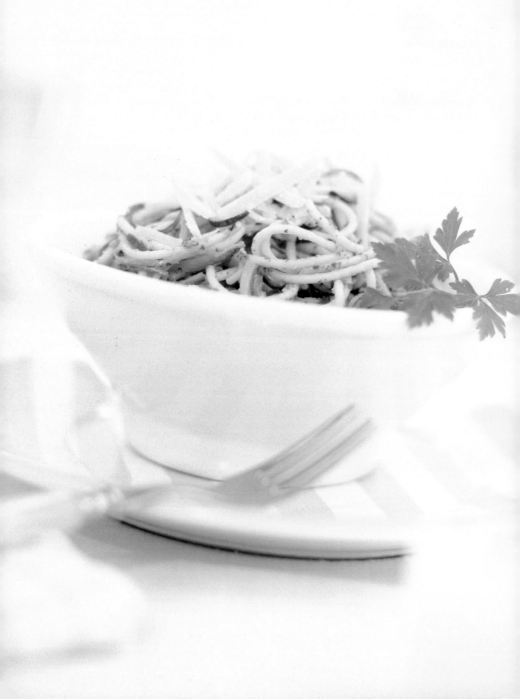

6 Menu suggestions

The freedom and flexibility of calorie counting mean that there's no need for elaborate or complicated menu plans. However, guidelines can be useful, especially when it comes to snacks. In this chapter you'll find some basic ideas; the recipes for some of them can be found in chapter 7.

Menu suggestions

It is vital to eat three nutritious evenly spaced-out meals a day. If you skip any you will feel starving and willpower could wobble. Eat healthy snacks between meals to stave off temptation.

Breakfast

Remember that this is an important meal and try not to miss out on it. Here are some suggestions; almost all are very quick to prepare. Butter toast very lightly.

• 200g unsweetened apple purée with two slices of wholemeal toast: 270 calories.
• A small boiled egg, with two slices of wholemeal toast: 280 calories.
• 30g grapenuts with a few sultanas, three small dried apricots, chopped, and 100g low-fat natural yoghurt: 215 calories.
• Porridge made with 30g dry weight of porridge oats and a few sultanas, cooked in water: 125 calories.
• A small can of baked beans and two slices of wholemeal toast: 305 calories.
• Two large slices of wholemeal toast and Marmite: 210 calories.
• Two grilled tomatoes, mushrooms cooked in a little olive oil, 2 small slices of wholemeal toast: 290 calories.

And some which can vary in calories more:
• Low-fat natural yoghurt made into a smoothie by blending it together with fresh berries.
• No-added-sugar muesli with chopped fresh fruit; measure carefully and don't forget to count the milk.
• Grapefruit and orange pieces; two slices of wholemeal toast.

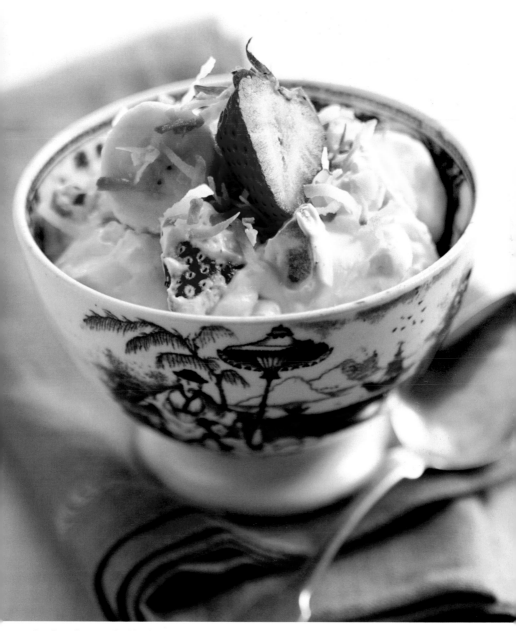

Greek yoghurt can be high in calories; choose no-fat versions.

Lunch

Adding green salad to dishes is an excellent way of increasing the amount you eat at minimal calorie cost, and salad leaves can be adventurous. Don't, however, buy packs which include high-fat, high-calorie dressings or calorific added ingredients like croûtons. Dress the salad yourself, or try it without a dressing – which is perfectly acceptable if the rest of your meal is strongly flavoured.

All of the following lunch suggestions come in at between 300 and 350 calories. Page references are given for the recipes in chapter 7.

• Two-egg mushroom or tomato omelette cooked in 1 teaspoon olive oil, with a large green salad and followed by fresh fruit.

• Tomato and red pepper soup (see page 127), two oatcakes and an eighth of a Camembert; a small piece of fresh fruit.

• Lentil, onion and coriander soup (see page 126) followed by no-fat Greek yoghurt with a teaspoon of honey and a few sultanas mixed in.

• Grilled goat's cheese on mushrooms (see page 132) followed by fresh fruit salad.

• Lebanese bread salad (see page 130) with a roast skinless chicken breast (seasoned with herbs and black pepper and cooked in the oven for 30 minutes at 200°C/gas mark 6 using half a teaspoon of olive oil to prevent sticking).

• Tsatsiki made with no-fat Greek yoghurt, chopped cucumber and garlic, served with a wholemeal pitta.

• Tunisian eggs (see page 136) with a large green salad, followed by fresh fruit.

• Salade Niçoise made with raw vegetables including tomatoes, lettuce, cucumber, green beans and

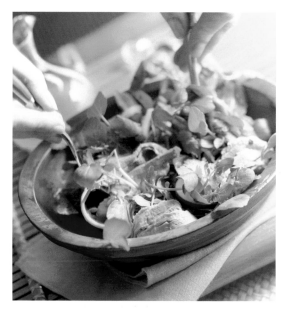

Add a variety of leaves to your salads, such as watercress, rocket, lamb's lettuce and fresh herbs.

spring onion, a small tin of tuna and a hard-boiled egg, decorated with a few anchovies drained of their oil and blotted on kitchen paper.

• Tuna and chive pâté (see page 146) used as filling for a wholemeal roll, or served with crudités and a slice of wholemeal bread.

• Cold oriental chicken (see page 148) with salad, followed by fresh fruit or a low-fat yoghurt.

• Smoked salmon with lemon and two small slices of wholemeal bread.

Main meals

Be careful when choosing meal accompaniments other than salad or plain green vegetables. Watch the quantity you serve and don't forget to add the calorie value to your total. You'll find calorie counts for the recipes in chapter 7 on the page where each recipe appears.

need to know

Sandwich tips

When choosing sandwich ingredients, avoid high-calorie spreads like mayo. Keep it as plain as you can – tomato salad, cold beef or chicken salad, smoked salmon – and go for wholemeal bread (unbuttered if possible).

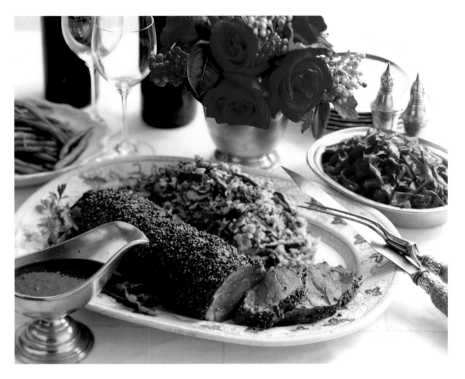

Watch out for the gravy with roast meats; they can bump up the calorie total significantly.

• Valpolicella risotto (see page 137) with green salad.

• Keralan prawn curry (see page 141) with a cucumber raita made using low-fat natural yoghurt, and a wholemeal pitta.

• Cold roast chicken breast, salad and 225g new potatoes: about 350 calories.

• Warm lentil, bacon and spinach salad (see page 133) with a wholemeal roll.

• Roast salmon with courgettes (see page 140).

• Spicy chickpea, spinach and aubergine casserole (see page 138) with simple chicken or lamb kebabs (remove all the visible fat before grilling).

• Smoked haddock fishcakes (see page 142) with a large green leaf and tomato salad.

• Vegetable stir-fry, cooked in as little oil as possible, served with 40g dry weight brown Basmati rice: about 300 calories.

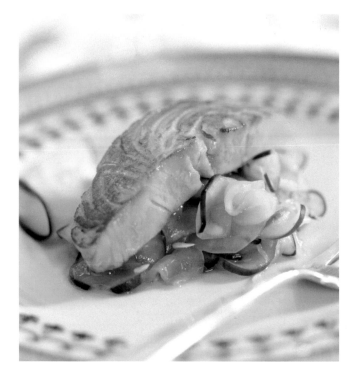

Fish is full of nutrients, and steaming – or baking in a foil parcel – will retain more than other cooking methods.

• Garlic prawns: 225g king prawns, cooked in a teaspoon of olive oil with plenty of chopped garlic and chilli, served with a wholemeal roll and a green salad: about 450 calories.
• Sirloin steak: 200g of good-quality beef with visible fat removed, served with mustard, and a large green salad dressed with a little olive oil and lemon juice: 400-450 calories

Desserts

Always remember that puddings are optional! Fresh fruit is usually the best bet, and there are some fruit-based desserts in the recipe chapter (see pages 151-5). Here are some other suggestions for a sweet ending to your meal.
• A small meringue nest, filled with a few chopped strawberries or raspberries and a level tablespoon of low-fat crème fraîche: 130 calories.

Cherries contain ellagic acid, a phytochemical that blocks the action of cancer-causing cells.

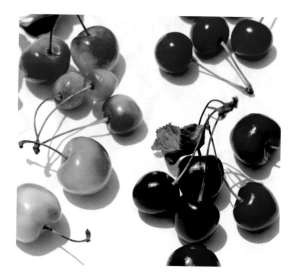

• 20g of high-cocoa-content dark chocolate and black coffee: 115 calories.

• Slices of ripe canteloupe melon: half an average one is about 200g and 38 calories.

• 150g no-fat Greek yoghurt with a teaspoon of clear honey and three almonds, chopped and dry-roasted in a non-stick pan: 149 calories.

• A large ripe mango, chopped and drizzled with a teaspoon of clear honey: 93 calories.

• A small banana, chopped and mixed with two chopped dates and a tablespoon of low-fat crème fraîche: 140 calories.

Here are some where the calories will vary more:

• A drink made from chopped, peeled and deseeded watermelon, blended and then added to low-calorie dry ginger ale – don't blend them at the same time or you'll have a flood; mix them together afterwards.

• An exotic fresh fruit salad made with mango, pineapple, kiwi fruit and whatever else you can find, like fresh lychees and pomegranate seeds.

- A small helping of vanilla ice cream with fresh fruit.
- Sliced pears with raspberry purée.

Snacks

Fresh fruit is an excellent option but steer snacking away from high-fat, high-sugar, high-calorie foods.

- A 125g pot of low-fat yoghurt: 70 calories.
- Five small dried apricots: 75 calories.
- 100g grapes: 60 calories.
- 200g cherries: 96 calories.
- One crispbread with cottage cheese: about 90 calories.
- Raw vegetable crudités with low-fat soft cheese: about 70-100 calories.
- A small slice of wholemeal toast with Marmite: about 95 calories.
- Five almonds and a peach: 110 calories.
- A bran or black pepper oatcake thinly spread with smooth peanut butter: about 95 calories.
- An apple and 25g Edam: about 145-165 calories.
- A plain oatcake with two blotted anchovy fillets on it (or a little anchovy paste): about 90 calories.
- A couple of quartered tomatoes with some ground black pepper to dip them in: about 60 calories.
- A small bowl of low-sugar jelly: about 20 calories.
- A fruit and vanilla ice cream lolly: 75-90 calories.
- 10g dark chocolate (about 55 calories), for those moments when you must...

Finally, don't forget that calorie counting can be infinitely adaptable. If you want to enjoy a glass of wine with your Valpolicella risotto, then forgo your evening (or afternoon) snack. The chances are that you won't need it anyway.

want to know more?

- Try slimming clubs, such as Weightwatchers, if you need support.
- Slimming magazines give recipes with their nutritional values, but note that some of them are owned by food companies and may recommend processed foods.
- There are lots of low-calorie and calorie-counted recipes online, changing all the time. Google both options, and see what you get.

websites

- www.weightloss resources.co.uk/recipes
- www.sainsburys .co.uk/food
- www.bbc.co.uk/ food/recipes
- www.watercress.co.uk
- www.eggrecipes.co.uk.
- www.weightwatchers .co.uk
- www.caloriecounting .co.uk

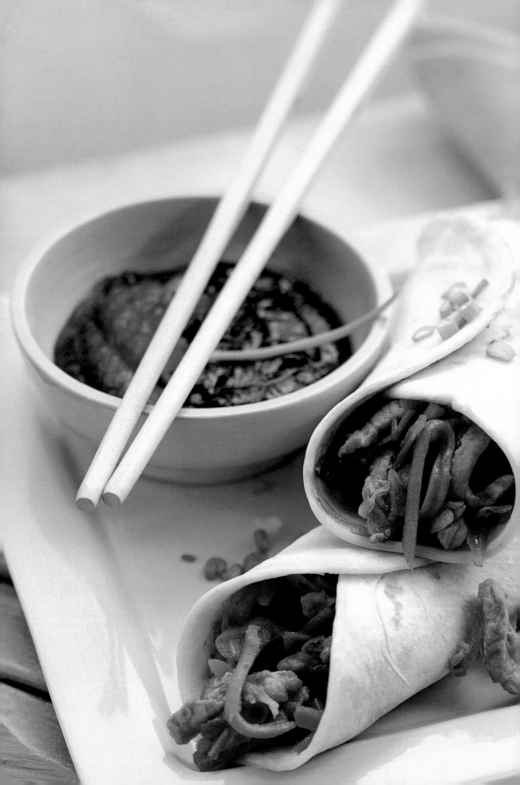

7 Recipes

All recipes in this chapter serve four; the calorie values given are for one serving of the dish itself and do not include any accompaniment you might choose to serve with it. They are suitable for non-dieters, who could easily accompany them with extras like potatoes or bread if they wished to do so. Accurate weighing and measuring is essential. All spoon measures are level; a teaspoon is 5ml and a tablespoon is 15ml.

Lentil, onion and coriander soup

A rich, flavoursome soup that is high in fibre yet low in calories. Perfect for lunch on a dreary winter day.

Ingredients:

125g green lentils
1 tsp olive oil
2 medium red onions, chopped
1 clove of garlic, finely chopped
A pinch of cinnamon
900ml water or vegetable stock
A large handful of fresh coriander
   leaves, chopped
Juice of half a lemon
Salt and black pepper

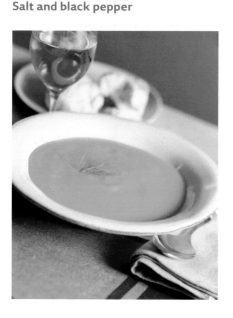

Rinse the lentils well and check them for any small stones.

Warm the olive oil in a large non-stick saucepan. Add the onions and cook gently until soft; try not to let them brown too much. Just before they are fully soft add the garlic, stir and cook for another couple of minutes.

Add the rinsed lentils and the cinnamon and stir to combine them thoroughly. Then add the water or vegetable stock and simmer until the lentils soften – the time this takes will depend on how fresh they are, but should be about 30 minutes. When they are almost soft, but still have a bit of bite, add the coriander leaves, keeping some back for a garnish, and the lemon juice.

Cook a little longer until the lentils are completely soft. Check the seasoning, adding salt and black pepper if you wish, and serve, garnished with a few coriander leaves.

Calories per portion: 136

Tomato and red pepper soup

There's no need to thicken soup with flour or add high-calorie extras like cream when you cook it with beans.

Ingredients:
60g dried cannellini beans
1 tsp olive oil
1 medium onion, chopped
1 carrot, chopped
1 stick of celery, chopped
2 red peppers, deseeded and
   chopped
1 clove of garlic, chopped
400g tinned tomatoes
800ml water or vegetable stock
A handful of fresh coriander or
   basil, chopped
Salt and black pepper

Soak the cannellini beans overnight. Drain and rinse them, put them in fresh water and bring to the boil. Cook for 10 minutes and then lower the heat and cook for 15 minutes.

Meanwhile, warm the oil in a large non-stick pan. Add the chopped onion, carrot and celery and cook gently in the oil until they begin to soften, then add the red peppers and the garlic. Stir the ingredients together and let them cook a little longer. Drain the cannellini beans and add them too. Finally add the tomatoes and their juices, and the liquid (filling the empty tomato can twice will give you the right amount, plus you'll get all the tomato juice).

Cook for 20 minutes until the beans and vegetables are tender, then add a handful of fresh coriander or basil. Check for seasoning and add a little salt and black pepper. Blend the soup, retaining some texture, then reheat it briefly before serving.

Calories per portion: 128

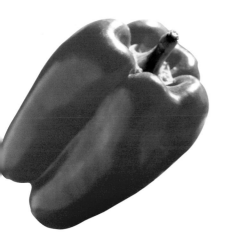

Carrot and ginger soup

A perennial favourite, this tasty soup makes an elegant first course for a dinner party.

Ingredients:
A sliver of butter, not more than
10g
1 medium onion, chopped
700g carrots, chopped
A 3cm cube of fresh ginger, grated
Salt and black pepper
900ml water or vegetable stock

Melt the butter in a non-stick pan with a lid, or use a casserole that can go on the hob. Add the chopped onion and cook gently, without letting it brown, until it is soft. Add the carrots, ginger and a little salt, stir thoroughly and cover tightly.

Cook the vegetables gently for about 10 minutes until everything has softened, but check during this time to make sure they are not browning. When they are ready add a little black pepper, then add the water or stock and cook for another 10–15 minutes. Blend the soup until smooth and then serve. If it is thicker than you want, add some more hot water and reheat before serving.

Calories per portion: 100

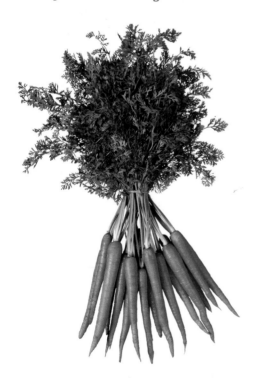

must know

Spice it up

If you like the taste, some ground coriander or cumin could be added with the carrots. This soup is very flexible.

Leek, potato and saffron soup

A hearty, satisfying soup that is made special by the addition of the saffron strands.

Ingredients:

650ml vegetable stock or water
250g leeks, chopped and rinsed well
1 small onion, chopped
200g potatoes, washed and chopped, but not peeled
2 cloves of garlic, chopped
A pinch of saffron strands
150ml hot water
Black pepper
Half a 400g tin of flageolet beans, drained and rinsed

Put the vegetable stock in a large pan and heat it until it is just about to boil. Add the leeks, onion, potatoes and garlic, reduce the heat and simmer for 10 minutes. Dissolve the saffron strands in the hot water and add to the pan. Grind black pepper into the soup generously and continue to cook; after another 5 minutes add the flageolet beans. Cook for 5 minutes and then blend the soup roughly – this is a country soup, and shouldn't be a completely smooth purée. Check for seasoning, adding more black pepper at this point, and some salt if you wish. Reheat and serve.

Calories per portion: 101

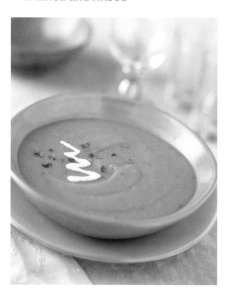

must know

Bean salad

Use the rest of the beans to make a salad with tuna, chopped red onion, tomato and olives. Serve on a bed of lettuce, and mix in other beans if you wish.

Lebanese bread salad

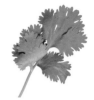

There are lots of versions of this traditional salad (one even includes beetroot) but this goes back to the original.

Ingredients:
2 wholemeal pitta breads
1 clove of garlic, halved
120g rocket
1 green pepper, deseeded and
  chopped
1 cucumber, chopped
6 spring onions, chopped
1 small red onion, finely chopped
8 medium tomatoes, deseeded
  and chopped
8 olives, chopped (optional)
A handful each of fresh mint, fresh
  parsley and fresh coriander, all
  chopped
Juice of 1 lemon
1 tsp olive oil
Salt and black pepper

Brown the pittas under the grill until they are crisp; allow them to become cool enough to handle and break them up, splitting them into pieces not bigger than 2cm.

Rub a big serving bowl with the cut surfaces of the garlic, and add the rocket, green pepper, cucumber, spring onions and red onion, tomatoes, olives and herbs. Mix well. Then put the lemon juice and the olive oil in a screw-top jar with a secure lid, seal it and shake well to make a dressing.

Traditionally the bread was added to the dressing at this stage and left to soak up the flavours for an hour or so before it was mixed with the rest of the salad. Today many people prefer to dress the salad with the oil and lemon mixture, tossing it well, and then add the crunchy pitta bread croûtons, mixing them in at the last minute. Try whichever method appeals to you.

Calories per portion: 156

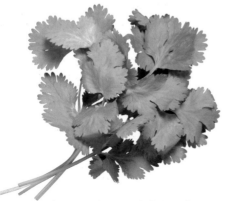

Pear and Roquefort salad

This is a classic combination of sweet and salty flavours, and several different textures, making it a salad with a difference.

Ingredients:

2 medium to large pears, ripe but not very soft

1 tbsp cider vinegar

2 tsp olive oil

Black pepper

200g strong-tasting salad leaves (like rocket, radicchio, baby spinach or endive), washed and drained

100g Roquefort cheese

20g chopped walnuts

must know

To serve

For a light lunch, accompany this with a slice of wholemeal or sourdough bread, unbuttered – the better the bread, the better the taste, and you won't need the butter.

Cut the pears into quarters and remove the cores; slice them finely and place in a large bowl. Put the cider vinegar and olive oil into a screw-top jar, grind in a generous quantity of black pepper, seal the jar well and shake it vigorously to mix the dressing. Pour this over the pears and turn them gently so that they are well covered; this will help to prevent them from discolouring.

Put the washed salad leaves into the same bowl, and stir them around gently in the dressing. Then put a pile of leaves and pear slices on each plate, making sure the pear slices are evenly shared, and crumble the Roquefort over each salad. Scatter a few chopped walnuts over the top of each one, and serve immediately.

Calories per portion: 173

Grilled goat's cheese on mushrooms

The powerful taste of the goat's cheese is balanced by the strong-flavoured salad and a dressing that packs a punch.

Ingredients:

4 large flat mushrooms, peeled

3 tsp olive oil, or a spray and 2 tsp oil

2 rounds of goat's cheese, about 1cm deep – approx 100g each

100g strong-tasting salad leaves, or a mixture of cos lettuce and rocket, washed and drained

1 small red onion, chopped in rings

2 ripe tomatoes, sliced

1 tbsp good balsamic vinegar

Salt and black pepper

must know

Oil spray

If you use an oil spray the calorie count will be lower. They can be found fairly easily and you can add the oil of your choice rather than relying on supermarket versions which often don't contain the healthiest oils.

Trim the stalks as close to the underside of the mushrooms as possible. Heat the grill, and cover the grid of the grill pan in foil. Put the mushrooms on the foil underside downwards, and spray with the olive oil, or put a couple of drops on each one, then grill them until they begin to colour slightly. Remove the pan from the grill and turn the mushrooms over.

Slice each round of goat's cheese into two – this is easier if your knife is really sharp and wiped so that it is slightly damp. Put a round of cheese on each mushroom and drizzle a little olive oil on each round. Replace under the grill. When the goat's cheese begins to bubble and then colour, it is ready.

While you wait for it to cook, put salad leaves on each plate, spreading them out, then scatter with onion rings and sliced tomatoes. Drizzle the salad with the balsamic vinegar. When the mushrooms and goat's cheese are ready, put one on each plate on top of the salad leaves. Season and serve immediately.

Calories per portion: 216

Warm lentil, bacon and spinach salad

Serve this on individual plates to ensure that everyone gets their fair share of the bacon.

Ingredients:
200g dried green or puy lentils
1 clove of garlic, halved
225g baby spinach leaves, washed
and rinsed
4 rashers of back bacon
2 tomatoes, chopped
1 red onion, chopped
A handful of mint leaves

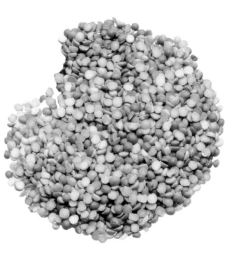

Check the lentils for little stones, wash them in a sieve, put them in fresh water and bring to the boil. Cook until just soft; how long this takes will depend on how fresh the lentils are, but it shouldn't exceed 25–30 minutes. Remove from the heat but leave them in their cooking water.

Rub four plates with the cut side of the garlic. Remove any tough-looking stems from the spinach and divide between the plates. Put the bacon under the grill, using the rack of the grill pan so the fat will drip away as the bacon cooks. Cook it well, and when it is nearly crispy drain the lentils, rinsing them with some boiling water. Put them in a clean bowl, add the tomatoes, onion and mint leaves and stir well to combine.

Spoon the lentil mixture on top of the spinach. Remove the bacon from the grill and blot any excess fat with kitchen paper, then chop a rasher over each plate of salad and serve immediately.

Calories per portion: 239

Hot beef stir-fry

This oriental-style stir-fry is easy to prepare when you get in from work and doesn't seem like 'diet food' at all.

Ingredients:

For the marinade:

Juice of 1 lime

2 tsp soy sauce

500g lean beef steak, cut into fine
  strips

2 tsp sesame oil

2 yellow peppers, deseeded and
  chopped

10 spring onions, chopped

1 medium red onion, chopped

100g mangetout, chopped into
  pieces about 2cm long

2cm cube of ginger, finely chopped

1 small chilli, deseeded and
  chopped

2 cloves of garlic, finely chopped

Put the lime juice and soy sauce in a bowl and stir them together. Add the beef strips, stirring to ensure all pieces have been in contact with the marinade, then cover and chill for at least 30 minutes. (Use this time to prepare the rest of the ingredients.)

Heat a non-stick wok and add the sesame oil. When it is really hot, remove the beef strips from the marinade using a slotted spoon and add them to the wok. Discard the marinade. Cook the beef, stirring, until it is medium rare. Remove it from the wok, again using a slotted spoon. You may find that the meat gives off a lot of liquid; reduce this down by boiling until you have about 2 tablespoons.

Add the peppers, spring onions, red onion and mangetout and cook for 2 minutes; then add the ginger, chilli and garlic. Return the beef to the wok and cook, stirring, until all the vegetables are done – nicely crunchy but definitely cooked – and serve immediately.

Calories per portion: 240

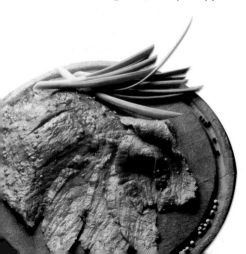

Tomato and rocket pasta

Some pastas are too high-calorie for a diet but this one is both low-cal and high-flavour.

Ingredients:

300g dried wholewheat spaghetti
2 tsp olive oil
2 garlic cloves, chopped
8 medium tomatoes, skinned, deseeded and chopped
2 tsp capers, rinsed and chopped
½ tsp dried oregano (or a handful of fresh, chopped)
Salt and black pepper
100g rocket, washed and roughly chopped

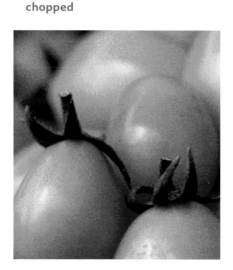

Bring a pan of water to the boil over a high heat and add the spaghetti. Cook according to the instructions on the pack.

Warm the oil in a non-stick frying pan, and when it is hot add the chopped garlic; stir it around and add the chopped tomatoes as it begins to colour. Stir well, and let the tomatoes cook for a couple of minutes, then add the capers and oregano. Continue to cook the mixture until the tomatoes begin to disintegrate – you may need to add a little water to prevent them from sticking; lower the heat if necessary. Grind some black pepper over them.

When the spaghetti is ready, drain it and return it to the pan. Put the tomato mixture and the rocket into the pan with the pasta and stir it around off the heat; the rocket will wilt a little. Check for seasoning, adding salt and more black pepper if you wish, and serve immediately.
Calories per portion: 305

Tunisian eggs

You can accompany these delicious baked eggs with a green salad and some kind of flat bread, such as pitta, if you wish.

Ingredients:

2 tsp olive oil

4 peppers – 1 red, 1 orange, 1 yellow, 1 green if possible – deseeded and chopped

1 medium onion, chopped

1 clove of garlic

4 medium tomatoes, deseeded and chopped

½ tsp paprika

½ tsp cayenne pepper

A dash of balsamic vinegar

Salt and black pepper

4 medium eggs

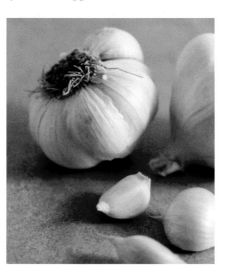

You will need an ovenproof dish or individual dishes which can be taken straight to the table. Preheat the oven to 200°C /gas mark 6.

Heat the oil in a large non-stick frying pan with a lid; put the chopped peppers and onion in the pan and stir them around. When they begin to sizzle loudly reduce the heat, add the garlic, stir and cover. Check every couple of minutes, and when the peppers are nicely soft put in the tomatoes and the spices. Add the balsamic vinegar, salt and black pepper, stir well and cover again.

Put the ovenproof dish or dishes in the oven to warm for a couple of minutes, and take the pepper mixture off the heat. Transfer the mixture to the warmed dish and make four indentations in it (or one in each individual dish) and carefully pour a raw egg into each; it is probably best to break the egg into another dish first, and then you can remove any stray pieces of shell. Cook in the oven for 8-10 minutes until the egg is just setting – ideally, the yolk should be just runny – and serve immediately.

Calories per portion: 185

Valpolicella risotto

This is a classic example of the old adage that the simplest dishes are often the best.

Ingredients:

2 tsp oil

3 small onions, peeled and finely chopped

1 fat clove of garlic

325g risotto rice

100ml Valpolicella, or similar red wine

Boiling water

Salt and black pepper

Fresh Parmesan, grated – optional

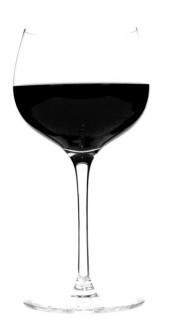

Boil a kettle. Heat the oil in a large non-stick frying pan with high sides and soften the onions and the garlic; don't let them brown. When they're beginning to go slightly transparent add the risotto rice and stir it around to coat it in what remains of the oil, but don't allow it to stick. After a minute or so, add about 300ml of hot water from the kettle, enough to almost cover the rice. Stir gently over a moderate heat until all the hot water has been absorbed, then add more (you may need to reboil the kettle).

Stir regularly, making sure all the grains are cooking, and continue adding more water and letting the rice absorb it until the grains are no longer hard, though they should still have a bit of bite. At this stage add the red wine – the risotto will turn a delicate pale pink – and stir until that has all been absorbed too.

Season to taste and serve immediately, with a green salad and Parmesan on the side: a small pinch, enough to lightly scatter the top of a serving of the risotto, will be about 5–10g.

Calories per portion: 343 (not including Parmesan)

Spicy chickpea, spinach and aubergine casserole

This makes a great accompaniment to plain grilled meat or poultry or is delicious by itself with wholemeal pitta.

Ingredients:

175g dried chickpeas

2 tsp olive oil

2 small onions, chopped

1 aubergine, chopped into 2cm cubes

2 garlic cloves, chopped

1 tbsp tomato purée

1 tsp harissa paste – or more if you like hot, spicy food

Juice and rind of 1 lemon

225g fresh spinach, washed and chopped

A large handful of fresh mint, chopped

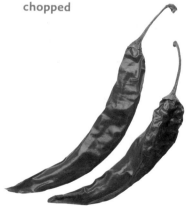

Soak the chickpeas overnight, drain and rinse them. Put them in a pan with fresh water and cook them until they are beginning to soften – how long this takes will depend on the age of the chickpeas as older ones take longer. Drain them, reserving the cooking liquid.

Warm a teaspoonful of olive oil in a heavy-bottomed pan or a casserole which can be used on the hob. Add the chopped onions and cook them gently for 10 minutes until they are soft. Meanwhile, warm the other teaspoonful of oil in a non-stick frying pan and cook the aubergine, also until it has browned. It will catch quickly at the end, so keep an eye on it.

Add the garlic, tomato purée and harissa to the onions and stir them together well. Allow them to cook for a minute or so, and then put the aubergine in too. Add a little of the cooking liquid from the chickpeas if the vegetables appear to be sticking. Stir them around for a minute or so, and then add the cooked chickpeas. Stir everything

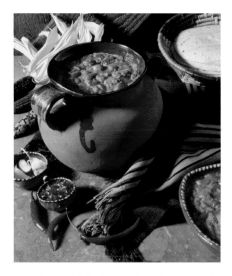

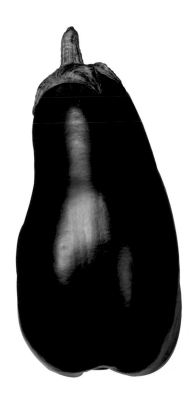

together, add the juice of the lemon and enough chickpea liquid to half-cover the ingredients. Cook for 15 minutes over a moderate-to-high heat; the liquid should start to reduce down.

Add the chopped spinach; you may need to do this in several batches, waiting while successive ones wilt before you can fit the next in the casserole. When it's all in, add some lemon rind, stir thoroughly and simmer for another 15 minutes. By now the liquid should be much reduced; stir in the mint and cook a little longer to reduce the liquid further. Serve hot.

Calories per portion: 204

Roast salmon with courgettes

This is a fantastic way to cook courgettes. The quantity may look excessive but they will reduce in the cooking.

Ingredients:
Half a lemon
4 salmon fillets, approximately
500g in total
4 medium to large courgettes
1 clove of garlic, chopped
Sliver of butter, not more than 10g
Salt and black pepper
4 tbsp low-fat crème fraîche

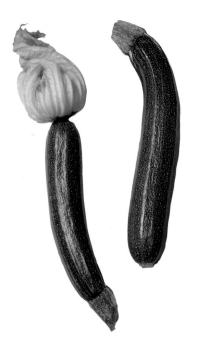

Preheat the oven to 200°C /gas mark 6. Squeeze the lemon into an ovenproof dish and put in the salmon fillets, turning them over in the juice and ending with them skin-side down. Cover the dish with foil and cook in the oven for 10 minutes.

Meanwhile, coarsely grate the courgettes. Crush the garlic and mix it with the grated courgette; add a little salt and black pepper.

Remove the foil from the salmon and replace it in the oven to continue cooking; how long this takes will depend on the thickness of the fillets – it could be between 5 and 10 minutes.

Put a large non-stick frying pan (or a non-stick wok) on the hob over a moderate heat and melt the sliver of butter in it. Add the grated courgettes and cook them gently – they should cook through rather than brown and it will not take long. When the salmon is ready, stir the crème fraîche into the courgettes and check for seasoning. Put a bed of courgette on each plate, and place a salmon fillet on top.
Calories per portion: 327

Keralan prawn curry

Serve this with a small portion of basmati rice. There are 103 calories in a 75g portion (about the size of a woman's fist).

Ingredients:

2 tsp sunflower or rapeseed oil

2 medium onions, chopped

2cm cube of fresh ginger, grated

2 cloves of garlic, finely chopped

4 medium tomatoes, deseeded and chopped

Juice of 1 small lemon

20g dessicated coconut

½ tsp ground turmeric

1 tsp ground coriander seeds

½ tsp cayenne pepper

150ml water

600g prawns

> **must know**
>
> **Turn up the heat**
>
> Traditionally, many Keralan dishes are very spicy. If you like hot food, then add a chopped chilli to the ginger, garlic and other ingredients when you make the paste.

Heat the oil in a large, heavy-bottomed pan. Add the chopped onion and cook, stirring, for 7–8 minutes until it is brown and beginning to soften. Remove from the heat.

Put the ginger, garlic, tomatoes, lemon juice and dessicated coconut in a blender or food processor and process until you have a rather liquid paste. Put the onion pan back on the heat and add the ginger mixture; stir it well. Then add the turmeric, coriander and cayenne, and finally the water. Bring to the boil, then lower the heat and cover, simmering gently for 10 minutes or so. Check to make sure it isn't catching and add more liquid if it is.

Increase the heat, bringing the sauce back up to the boil. Add the prawns, stirring them in gently, and cook them at this high temperature, still stirring gently, for about 5 minutes. The sauce should be thick; add more water if you prefer a thinner one. Serve immediately.

Calories per portion: 254

Smoked haddock fishcakes

It's worth taking the time to make your own fishcakes as they are worlds away from shop-bought ones.

Ingredients:

500g fresh smoked haddock fillets

500g new potatoes

15g butter

Black pepper

A handful of chopped fresh chives

1 large egg, beaten

15g fine wholemeal flour

30g wholemeal breadcrumbs

1 tbsp sunflower or rapeseed oil

must know

Haddock

Try to find undyed smoked haddock. It is much paler than the bright orange fillets and is becoming much more widely available (and cheaper) than it was. The taste is definitely superior.

You can either cook the fish in a pan or in the microwave (which minimizes the smell). For the first method, put the whole fillets in a large pan, add water to almost cover and poach over a gentle heat until the fish flakes easily – about 5 minutes. To microwave, put the fillets in a microwave-proof dish, add water, cover with appropriate cling film and puncture the film in several places. Microwave until cooked, following the instructions for your particular oven – at 800W it should take about 3 minutes. Let the fish cool on a plate, reserving the cooking liquid.

Boil the new potatoes in their skins until they are soft. Chop them roughly, add the butter and black pepper and mash them, using a couple of spoonfuls of the liquid from the fish. Keep the mash fairly dry; it should hold together but not be sloppy.

Now add the fish, flaking it well, and the chopped chives. Stir and then add most of the beaten egg – reserve about a third – and stir again. Put the mixture into a bowl and chill in the fridge for at least 30 minutes.

Cover a baking tray in foil or baking paper, and remove the fish mixture from the fridge. Sprinkle a small quantity of flour on a board. Using a spoon, divide the mixture into eight balls, each about the size of a satsuma, then rub your hands on the flour and form the balls into fat fishcakes, flattening each one a little. Brush each lightly with the reserved beaten egg, dab with breadcrumbs on both sides and put them on the baking tray. Chill them again, also for at least 30 minutes.

To cook, put the oil in a large non-stick frying pan and heat it; when it is hot slide the fishcakes in one by one and cook gently, turning them over to do both sides.

Serve with a green salad and a fresh tomato salsa made with chopped tomatoes and red onion.

Calories per portion (2 fishcakes): 342

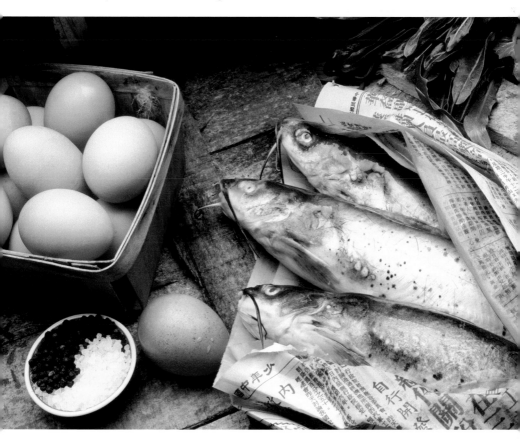

Baked fish and chips with tomato salsa

You may have thought this was one treat you would have to forgo on a diet: well, think again!

Ingredients:

800g 'old' potatoes – choose smaller ones

4 cod loins or chunky fillets, approx. 600g in total

1 lemon

2 tsp olive oil

4 tomatoes, chopped and deseeded

A handful each of fresh parsley and basil, chopped

Black pepper

2 tsp balsamic vinegar

Preheat the oven to 200°C / gas mark 6. Cut the unpeeled potatoes into slices not more than 1cm thick, and then cut the slices into chips also about 1cm wide or less. Put them in cold water.

Place the fish on a large piece of foil, pop a slice of lemon on each piece and squeeze the remaining lemon juice over. Lift the foil up and fold it together on the top, making a secure parcel; put this in an ovenproof dish. Making a long package rather than a square one, and using a long dish, will help you to fit everything in the oven.

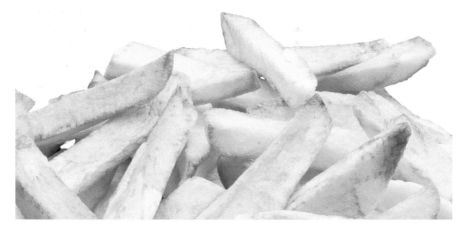

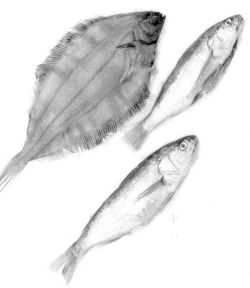

Drain the chips and dry them on a tea towel. Put them into a large plastic bag and add 2 tsp olive oil. Seal the bag carefully and then jiggle the chips about thoroughly to coat them in a light film of oil. Place the chips on a couple of non-stick baking trays, or ordinary ones lined with greaseproof paper, and space them out so there are gaps between them and none is touching the sides. Put the baking trays and the fish in the oven; cook for 10 minutes. Check the chips and turn them over. Bring out the dish with the fish in it and open the foil, exposing the top of the cod. Put it back in the oven with the chips for another 10 minutes.

Meanwhile, make the salsa: mix the chopped tomatoes and herbs in a bowl, add black pepper and balsamic vinegar, and stir everything together.

Check the fish is done and remove everything from the oven. Serve immediately, lifting the fish out of the foil with a slotted spoon so the juices are left behind (if necessary put it on some kitchen paper before transferring it to the plates). Serve with a green salad and a dish of salsa on the side.
Calories per portion, including salsa: 312

must know

Chips

The aim is to get both cod and chips ready at the same time. Choose medium-thickness fish if you can, but if your fish is very thick, put it in the oven before the potatoes; if it is thin, then add it after the potatoes have been in for 5 minutes. In calorie terms, there is enough leeway to add another small, 200g potato: if you do so, you shouldn't need to add any more oil, but you will have to adjust you daily calorie count...

Tuna and chive pâté

Supermarket-bought tuna pâté is usually chockful of fat and calories, but this low-cal version tastes every bit as good.

Ingredients:

2 x 80g tins of tuna in spring water
   or brine
200g extra light soft cheese
A little lemon juice
Tabasco sauce
Black pepper
A large handful of fresh chives,
   chopped

Drain the cans of tuna and flake the fish into a food processor or blender. Add the soft cheese and process briefly. Then add a small squeeze of lemon juice (being careful not to drop any pips in), two large dashes of Tabasco sauce, plenty of black pepper and the chives. Process until the mixture is smooth, tip into a bowl and chill, covered, for at least two hours.
Calories per portion: 99

This makes a good dip if you add a little more lemon juice and a 150g pot of low-fat natural yoghurt; for a firmer pâté add another tin of tuna. If you do either, don't forget to adjust the calorie count. The dip would have an overall count of 500, and the firmer pâté one of 460.

must know

Pâté and toast

Many patés and dips are so high in calories that it is impossible to eat them with anything other than raw vegetables if you are dieting. This one is low-calorie enough to serve with wholemeal toast. And if you are having paté with toast, then you don't really need butter – or a substitute – on the toast as well.

Chicken with mushrooms

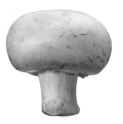

An ideal family supper that could be served with new potatoes and some steamed green veg on the side.

Ingredients:

1 tsp olive oil

2 cloves of garlic, chopped

4 skinless chicken breasts

500g button mushrooms, chopped

2 tomatoes, skinned and chopped

½ tsp dried oregano, or Italian mixed herbs

120ml dry white wine

Salt and black pepper

Warm the oil in a large non-stick pan with a lid. When it is hot, add the chopped garlic and stir. Then put in the chicken breasts and turn them over in the oil and cook for a few minutes – don't let them really brown, though: they should be slightly golden all over.

Add the mushrooms, tomatoes and dried herbs to the pan, followed by the wine, and stir everything together. At first there doesn't seem to be much liquid, but this soon increases as the mushrooms and tomatoes begin to cook. Simmer, and after about 15 minutes, check the liquid and stir again; if the liquid is reducing significantly, cover the pan and lower the heat a little. Add a little salt and black pepper if you wish at this stage. Cook for another 15 minutes, stirring occasionally to make sure nothing sticks; some liquid should remain. Check the seasoning, and serve immediately.

Calories per portion: 218

must know

Dried mushrooms

Add a few dried mushrooms, such as ceps, for extra depth of flavour. Though they are higher in calories than fresh mushrooms, they are very light – 5g would be fine here and would only add 12 calories. Soak them in warm water for at least an hour before using, rinse well and discard the soaking water. Pat dry, chop and add with the button mushrooms.

Oriental chicken with lemon, ginger, garlic and soy

Chicken can sometimes be dry, but not when cooked in this zingy marinade. Serve hot, cold, or sliced in sandwiches.

Ingredients:
4 skinless chicken breasts
Juice of 1 lemon
2cm cube of fresh ginger
2 cloves of garlic
2 tbsp light soy sauce
2 tbsp dry sherry or vermouth

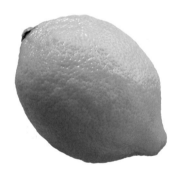

Rinse the chicken breasts and pat them dry. Put the lemon juice in a bowl large enough to hold the chicken; grate the ginger and garlic into the bowl, discarding any chunks left as you get to the end of the piece of ginger or cloves of garlic. Add the soy sauce and the dry sherry or vermouth, then add the chicken pieces. Turn them around in the liquid, making sure they have all been in contact with it, then cover the bowl and refrigerate for at least four hours and not longer than twelve hours.

Preheat the oven to 190°C /gas mark 5. Remove the chicken pieces from the bowl and put them in an ovenproof dish. Pour the liquid from the bowl over them, scraping any lingering pieces of garlic or ginger onto the chicken. Bake the chicken breasts for 35-40 minutes until thoroughly cooked, turning it over once. Some of the liquid should still remain.

If you want to serve it hot, you could accompany it with boiled rice and steamed mangetout and you can spoon some of the liquid over the rice.

This is also extremely good cold, a home-made version of the bright red 'Chinese chicken' found in supermarkets but without any artificial colouring. Remove the chicken breasts from the cooking dish and put them on a plate, discard any remaining liquid and refrigerate once cold. Eat them within 24 hours.

Calories per portion (one chicken breast): 172

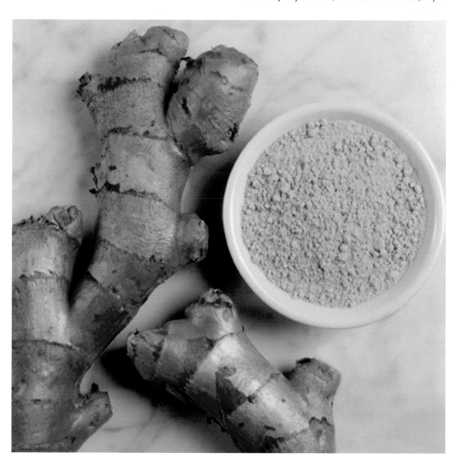

Sautéed pork fillet with herbs and white wine

This quick-cook supper dish will satisfy dieters and non-dieters alike.

Ingredients:

750g pork fillet

2 tsp olive oil

2 bay leaves

A handful of fresh rosemary leaves

Black pepper

100ml dry white wine

must know

Cuts of pork

Pork is often thought of as being fatty, but pork fillet or tenderloin is lower in calories than a lot of other meats, and cubes of pork fillet also work well in stir-fries or casseroles.

Rinse and dry the pork fillets. Cut them into fine strips not longer than 5cm and not thicker than 1cm; they should all be about the same size. Heat the olive oil in a large non-stick frying pan; add the bay leaves and turn them in the oil a couple of times. Then add the pork fillet strips and the rosemary and cook, stirring to make sure the pork doesn't stick.

Continue cooking until it is brown on both sides, which happens quite suddenly. Remove the bay leaves now if they are beginning to burn; otherwise discard them just before serving. Grind black pepper over the pork and pour the wine into the pan. Cook, boiling the wine until it has reduced almost completely. Serve immediately.

This is good with a tomato and red onion salad, which cuts the richness of the pork, as well as a simple green salad. Non-dieters could accompany it with some fresh pasta.

Calories per portion: 315

Baked oranges with cinnamon and Cointreau

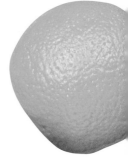

Accompany this tangy orange dish with some crème fraîche or no-fat Greek yoghurt if you wish.

Ingredients:
4 large, juicy oranges
1 tsp cinnamon
1 tbsp dark brown sugar
4 tsp Cointreau

must know

Serving suggestion

You can use one large dish, but it is easier to share the oranges – and their juice – evenly if you use four. A single dish could always be taken straight to the table, though.

You need four ovenproof dishes. Preheat the oven to 200°C /gas mark 6. Peel the oranges carefully, removing as much pith as possible, but being careful not to dig into the orange itself: it helps if you scrape the pith away gently with a very sharp knife.

Using the same sharp knife, cut the oranges into slices about 3mm thick and put each sliced orange in an ovenproof dish. Sprinkle a little cinnamon over the top of each one, then do the same with the brown sugar. Finally, drip a teaspoon of Cointreau into each dish and cover the individual dishes tightly with foil.

Bake in the oven for 15 minutes until the oranges are warm; they should not be piping hot. Serve immediately, turning them onto individual plates or bowls, pouring any juice over them.
Calories per portion: 110

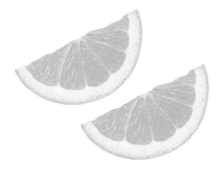

Baked peaches with amaretti biscuits

Try this for a summer dinner party when peaches are sweet and plentiful, but don't overdo the rum or you'll drown them.

Ingredients:

4 ripe peaches

8 soft amaretti biscuits

1 tbsp white rum

must know

Amaretti

Hard amaretti biscuits may be easier to get hold of than soft ones. If you are using hard ones, allow the biscuit and rum mixture to stand for a little to soften – make it before you halve the peaches. You may find you need a little more rum.

Preheat the oven to 190°C /gas mark 5. You need an ovenproof dish large enough to hold eight peach halves in one layer.

Cut each peach in half and remove the stones (cut through the peach to the stone and then twist one half away from the other). The stone will have to be cut out of the other half; don't worry too much about neatness. Place the peaches cut side uppermost in a large ovenproof dish.

Crush the amaretti biscuits between your fingers into a small bowl or dish. Add a tablespoon of white rum and mix together. Spoon the amaretti and rum mixture into the gaps left by the stones in the peach halves. Bake in the oven for 15–20 minutes: the peaches should be very warm rather than very hot and the amaretti mixture should not be burnt. Serve immediately, with a little low-fat crème fraîche if you wish.

Calories per portion (two halves): 89

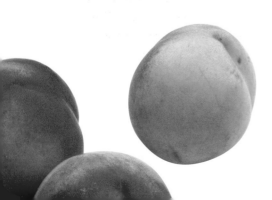

Refreshing mango and citrus salad

This unusual mixture of flavours and textures makes an interestingly different dessert.

Ingredients:
4 medium oranges
1 pink grapefruit
2 ripe mangoes
1 tbsp Cointreau
A small handful of fresh mint

must know

Mangoes

Mangoes are a great source of antioxidants, fibre and vitamin E. They aren't always ripe when you buy them, but will generally ripen at home – keep them in a warm kitchen until they give slightly in your hand.

Peel the oranges, removing as much pith as possible, then cut into segments. Remove the central pith and any pips carefully. Do the same with the grapefruit, though it may be easier to cut it into pieces first, and then slice the peel and pith off. Put all the pieces of citrus fruit in a large bowl.

Slice the mangoes and peel the slices, then cut the slices into pieces not larger than 2cm. Remove any fruit from around the stone – get as much as you can – and put the mango in the bowl with the oranges and grapefruit. Add the Cointreau and stir the fruit around until it is well mixed and has all been in contact with the Cointreau.

Stir in a few chopped leaves of fresh mint, garnish the fruit salad with some whole mint leaves and serve. This is best eaten on the day of preparation.

Calories per portion: 130

Plum compôte

The rich purply-red colour of this compôte looks spectacular if you serve it in a pretty glass dish.

Ingredients:
500g red plums
50ml water
1 tsp clear honey
1 tbsp brandy

must know

Plums

Red plums are a good choice because of the beta-carotene they contain, an important nutrient and antioxidant. They also give this dish its glorious colour; it wouldn't be the same with other plums. You can replace the brandy with water if you wish.

Wash the plums (unpeeled) and chop them into evenly sized pieces, discarding the stones. Put them into a non-stick pan over a moderate heat and add the water and the honey. Stir thoroughly.

As the liquid begins to boil the plums start to give up their juice. Add the brandy and continue cooking; the colour of the plums will change to a deep, garnet red. When most of the plums have begun to disintegrate remove the pan from the heat, put the plums into a bowl and allow them to cool.

These are good just as they are, served slightly warm. They also make a delicious sauce for good-quality ice cream and are lovely cold, served from the fridge and scattered with a few chopped almonds.
Calories per portion: 58

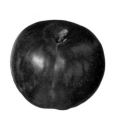

Apple and orange fool

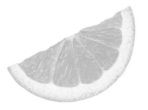

Rich, sweet and fruity yet only 100 calories per serving, this dessert is a dieter's dream.

Ingredients:

2 cooking apples, peeled, cored and cubed – about 400g
Juice and rind of 1 orange
1 tsp cinnamon
¼ tsp ginger
1 tbsp honey
300g no-fat Greek yoghurt

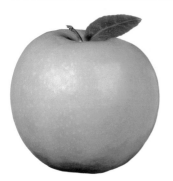

> **must know**
>
> **Fake cream**
>
> If you want a slightly richer taste, and can afford it in terms of calories, use a half-and-half mix of no-fat Greek yoghurt and low-fat crème fraîche.

Put the apples and orange juice in a non-stick pan over a moderate heat, reserving the orange rind; add the cinnamon, ginger and honey. Cook gently for about 10 minutes until the apple softens and disintegrates – stir continuously towards the end, breaking up the apples with the spoon. Add a little water if necessary but be cautious; you want the apples to absorb all the liquid.

Once the apples are thoroughly soft, remove the pan from the heat and let the mixture cool. When it is a lot cooler, put it into a food processor or blender and process until smooth, then transfer it into a bowl and put it in the fridge to chill for at least an hour.

Thoroughly mix the chilled purée with the yoghurt and spoon into serving dishes – wine glasses look good. Chill again for at least 30 minutes and serve garnished with fine strips of orange rind.
Calories per portion: 100

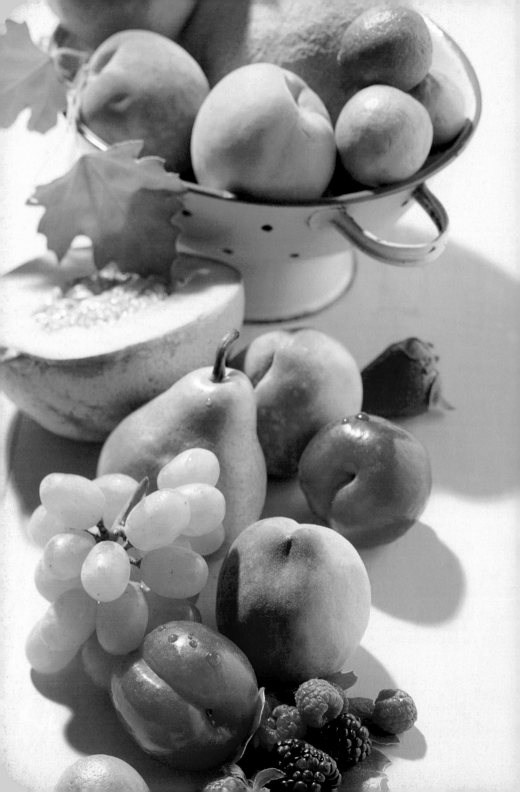

8 Listings

In this chapter you'll find the carbohydrate, fibre, calorie, protein and fat counts for average portions of some common foods. The listings are organized alphabetically by food type (i.e. Bakery, Beans, Breakfast cereals). Don't forget to check your actual portion size and do the sums if it is different from that mentioned here. The abbreviation n/a means that figures were not available for that particular item.

Bakery

Bread and bakery items can deal a fatal blow to any diet, so keep a careful note of how much you are actually eating. It's a good idea to stick to wholegrain bread and wheat products; they are slightly lower in calories and are much better for you than their refined-flour equivalents. If you use butter, remember to count the extra calories.

must know

Go Scandinavian

Cut 65–71 calories a time by turning ordinary sandwiches into open sandwiches – just remove the top slice of bread.

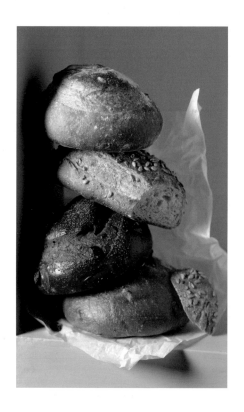

Food type	Carb (g)	Fibre (g)	Cal (kcal)	Pro (g)	Fat (g)
Brown bread, 1 slice	12.6	1.5	**62**	2.4	0.6
Croissant, each (70g)	30.3	2.2	**261**	5.8	13.8
Crumpet, each (50g)	15.9	1.5	**91**	3.0	0.4
Flour, 100g:					
wheat, white, breadmaking	70	3.1	**337**	11.0	1.4
wheat, white, plain	71	3.1	**336**	10.0	1.3
wheat, white, self-raising	72	2.0	**343**	11.0	1.2
wheat, wholemeal	58	9	**308**	14	2.2
French stick, 1 slice (2cm thick)	18.7	1.1	**88**	3.0	0.6
Granary bread, 1 slice	14.1	1.6	**71**	2.9	0.7
Naan, plain, half	31.2	1.8	**177**	4.9	4.5
Oatcakes, each:					
fine	6.3	0.9	**46**	1	2.2
organic	7.1	0.9	**42**	0.9	1.6
rough	6.4	8	**43**	1.2	1.8
traditional	5.8	0.8	**43**	1.1	1.7
Rye crispbread, each:					
dark rye	6.5	1.8	**31**	0.9	0.1
multigrain	5.7	1.7	**33**	1.1	0.6
original	6.7	1.7	**33**	1.1	0.1
Pitta bread, white, medium:	27.7	1.2	**128**	4.6	0.7
wholewheat	20.5	3.1	**114**	5.4	1.2
Rye bread, 1 slice	13.8	n/a	**66**	2.5	0.5
Sourdough bread, 1 slice	14.7	0.9	**78**	2.5	0.9
Stoneground wholemeal, 1 slice	11.8	2.2	**65**	2.9	0.7
White bread, 1 slice	13.9	0.8	**66**	2.4	0.5
Wholemeal, 1 slice	12.7	2.1	**66**	2.8	0.8

Beans, pulses and lentils

Beans and pulses are valuable sources of protein and fibre, as well as many other nutrients. They are all low in saturated fat and have a gentle effect on blood sugar. They can also be very tasty (and don't necessarily cause indigestion).

must know

Preparing beans

After soaking dried pulses, drain and rinse them thoroughly before you cook them - this will help to reduce any problems with flatulence. Some, like kidney beans, need to be boiled for 10 minutes before you turn the heat down.

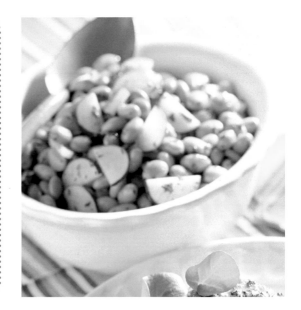

Food type	Carb (g)	Fibre (g)	Cal (kcal)	Pro (g)	Fat (g)
Aduki beans, 115g	25.9	n/a	**141**	10.7	0.2
Blackeyed beans, 115g	22.9	n/a	**133**	10.1	0.8
Bulgur wheat, dry, 100g	74	3.1	**357**	12	1.4
Butter beans:					
small can (200g)	21.8	9.6	**166**	12	0.8
dried, boiled (115g)	21.2	6	**118**	8.2	0.7
Chickpeas:					
small can (200g)	32.2	n/a	**230**	14.4	5.8
dried, boiled (115g)	20.9	n/a	**139**	9.7	2.4
Couscous, dry, 100g	72.5	2	**355**	23.5	1.9
Haricot beans, 115g					
dried, boiled	19.8	7	**109**	7.6	0.6
Lentils, 115g:					
green/brown, boiled	19.4	n/a	**121**	10.1	0.8
red, split, boiled	20.1	n/a	**115**	8.7	0.5
Red kidney beans:					
small can (200g)	27	12.8	**182**	16.2	1.0
boiled, 115g	20	n/a	**118**	9.7	0.6
Tofu (soya bean curd), 100g:					
steamed	0.7	–	**73**	8.1	4.2
fried	2.0	–	**261**	23.5	17.7

Breakfast cereals

Always eat breakfast or you may be tempted by high-calorie
snacks as your blood sugar goes into freefall later. Check that the
cereal you choose isn't packed with sugar, and be aware that some
weigh heavy – you may not get much for the calories they contain.

must know

Eat your grains

Several studies have
shown that people who
miss breakfast eat more
fatty food later in the day,
and are more likely to be
overweight.

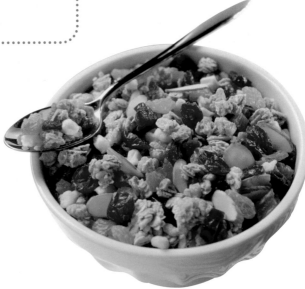

Food type	Carb (g)	Fibre (g)	Cal (kcal)	Pro (g)	Fat (g)
Bran flakes, 30g	19.8	4.5	**97**	3	0.6
Cornflakes, 30g:	23.4	0.9	**112**	2.1	0.3
High Fibre Bran, 40g	18.4	10.8	**112**	5.6	1.8
Muesli, 50g:	33	3.8	**182**	5	3.4
apricot	29.5	2.8	**142**	3.9	1.8
deluxe	28.1	5.8	**172**	5.4	5
high fibre	35.4	3	**158**	5.2	3
natural	31.5	4.3	**173**	4.8	3.1
organic	29.8	4.5	**177**	4.5	4.4
Swiss-style	36.1	n/a	**182**	4.9	3
with no added sugar	33.6	n/a	**183**	5.3	3.9
Oat bran flakes, 30g	20.1	0.6	**99**	3	0.6
Porridge (cooked), 100g:					
made with water	8.1	n/a	**46**	1.4	1.1
made with whole milk	12.6	n/a	**113**	4.8	5.1
Shredded wheat bisks, 30g:	20.3	3.5	**102**	3.5	0.8
bite-size	21	3.6	**105**	3.5	0.8
sugar coated	21.6	2.7	**105**	3	0.6
fruit-filled	20.6	2.7	**106**	2.5	1.5
Wheat bisks , 30g	20.4	3.0	**101**	3.5	0.6

Dairy products and eggs

These can be a danger area, so measure carefully, especially cheese. Be careful about choices, wean yourself off full-cream products, and include the calories from any milk added to hot drinks when you're calculating your daily total. Eggs are not the dietary demons they were once thought to be; nutritionally, they're extremely useful – see page 71 for more information.

Food type	Carb (g)	Fibre (g)	Cal (kcal)	Pro (g)	Fat (g)
Butter, see page 177					
Cheese, 25g:					
Brie	0.1	–	**76**	5.5	6
Cheddar, English	–	104	**6.4**	8.7	
Cheddar, vegetarian	Tr	–	**98**	6.4	8
Cheshire	–	–	**93**	5.8	7.8
Cottage cheese, plain	3.1	–	**101**	12.6	4.3
Cottage cheese, reduced fat	3.3	–	**79**	13.3	1.5
Edam	Tr	–	**85**	6.7	6.5
Feta	0.4	–	**63**	3.9	5.1
Lancashire	–	–	**93**	5.8	7.8
Roquefort	Tr	–	**89**	5.8	7.3
Stilton, blue	–	–	**103**	5.9	8.8
Wensleydale	–	–	**95**	5.8	8
Cream, 2 tbsp:					
fresh, double	0.5	–	**149**	0.5	16.1
fresh, single	0.7	–	**58**	1	5.7
fresh, whipping	0.8	–	**114**	0.6	12

Food type	Carb (g)	Fibre (g)	Cal (kcal)	Pro (g)	Fat (g)
Crème fraîche:					
full fat	0.7	–	**113**	0.7	12
half fat	1.3	–	**49**	0.8	4.5
Eggs, chicken, 1 medium:					
Raw, whole	Tr	–	**78**	6.5	5.8
Raw, white only	Tr	n/a	**17**	4.3	Tr
Raw, yolk only	Tr	n/a	**59**	2.8	5.3
Boiled	Tr	n/a	**76**	6.5	5.6
Eggs, duck, raw, whole	Tr	n/a	**84**	7.4	6.1
Milk, 250ml:					
cows', whole	11.3	n/a	**165**	8.3	9.8
semi-skimmed	11.8	–	**115**	8.5	4.3
skimmed	11	–	**80**	8.5	0.5
Soya milk, 250ml:					
sweetened	6.3	Tr	**108**	7.8	6
unsweetened	1.3	1.3	**65**	6	4
Yoghurt, 125g pot:					
Greek-style, plain	6	–	**166**	7.1	12.8
low-fat, plain	9.3	–	**70**	6	1.3
low-fat, fruit	17.1	0.4	**98**	5.3	1.4
whole milk, plain	9.8	–	**99**	7.1	3.8
whole milk, fruit	22.1	–	**136**	5	3.8

Drinks

Miscalculating – or forgetting – drink calories is a common problem. Double-check measures of alcohol, use low-calorie mixers and if you like fizzy drinks, change to low-calorie ones. You can forget about calories in tea or coffee when they are black or taken with lemon, but adding milk changes that (see page 165 for milk calories); cappuccinos and lattes can be very high-cal.

must know

Juicy fruit

Fruit juices can be high in calories, and also raise blood-sugar levels swiftly, so it is much better to eat the whole fruit. That way you will benefit from the fibre, too.

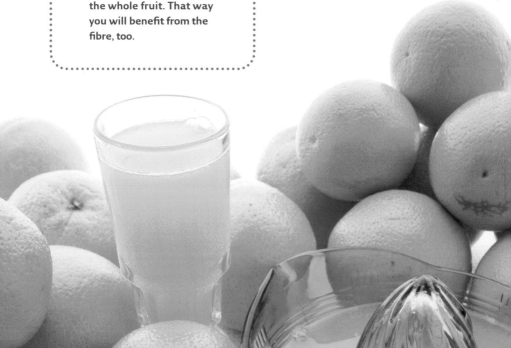

Food type	Carb (g)	Fibre (g)	Cal (kcal)	Pro (g)	Fat (g)
Alcoholic					
Beer, bitter, 500ml:	11.5	–	**160**	1.5	Tr
Brandy, 25ml	Tr	–	**56**	Tr	–
Cider, 500ml:					
dry	13	n/a	**180**	Tr	–
sweet	21.5	n/a	**210**	Tr	–
Gin, 25ml	Tr	–	**56**	Tr	–
Lager, bottled, 500ml	7.5	–	**145**	1.0	Tr
Orange liqueur, 25ml	n/a	n/a	**85**	n/a	–
Sherry, 25ml					
dry	0.4	n/a	**29**	0.1	–
medium	1.5	n/a	**29**	–	–
sweet	1.7	n/a	**34**	0.1	–
Vodka, 25ml	Tr	–	**56**	Tr	–
Whisky, 25ml	Tr	–	**56**	Tr	–
Wine, per small glass (125ml):					
red	0.3	n/a	**85**	0.1	–
rosé	3.1	n/a	**89**	0.1	–
white, dry	0.8	n/a	**83**	0.1	–
white, medium	3.8	n/a	**93**	0.1	–
white, sparkling	6.4	n/a	**93**	0.4	–
white, sweet	7.4	n/a	**118**	0.3	–
Non-alcoholic					
Apple juice, unsweetened, 250ml	24.8	n/a	**95**	0.3	0.3
Carrot juice, 250ml	14.3	–	**60**	1.3	0.3
Cranberry juice, 250ml	29.3	Tr	**123**	Tr	Tr
Orange juice, unsweetened, 250ml	22	n/a	**90**	1.3	0.3

Fish and seafood

Both fish and shellfish are great sources of protein and vitamins, and are low in fat. Oily fish like salmon and mackerel are high in omega-3 fatty acids, which are believed to be beneficial to health in all sorts of ways. Eating fish may help to reduce the risk of developing cardiovascular disease, so try and incorporate it in your diet – not fried fish in batter, though!

must know

Canned fish

Be wary of fish canned in oil. Even if you drain the oil away carefully, the fish will have absorbed some of it. Choose fish in brine or, even better, spring water.

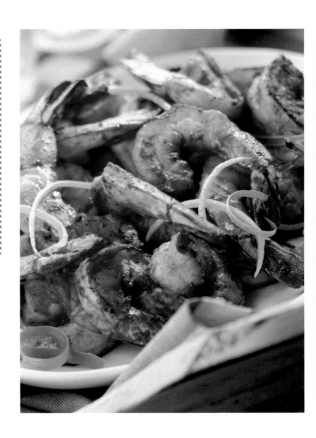

Food type	Carb (g)	Fibre (g)	Cal (kcal)	Pro (g)	Fat (g)
Cod:					
poached fillets, 100g	Tr	n/a	**94**	20.9	1.1
steaks, grilled, 100g	Tr	n/a	**95**	20.8	1.3
Haddock:					
smoked, steamed, 100g	–	n/a	**101**	23.3	0.9
steamed, 100g	–	n/a	**89**	20.9	0.6
Herring, raw, 100g	0	n/a	**190**	17.8	13.2
Kippers, grilled, 100g	–	n/a	**255**	20.1	19.4
Mackerel, 100g:					
raw	0	n/a	**220**	18.7	16.1
smoked	0	n/a	**354**	18.9	30.9
Plaice, steamed, 100g	–	–	**93**	18.9	1.9
Prawns:					
shelled, boiled, 100g	–	n/a	**99**	22.6	0.9
boiled, weighed in shells, 175g	–	–	**72**	15.1	1.2
king prawns, freshwater, 100g	–	n/a	**70**	16.8	0.3
tiger king, cooked, 100g	–	n/a	**61**	13.5	0.6
Salmon:					
grilled steak, 100g	–	n/a	**215**	24.2	13.1
smoked, 100g	–	n/a	**142**	25.4	4.5
steamed, flesh only, 100g	–	n/a	**194**	21.8	11.9
Trout:					
brown, steamed, 100g	–	–	**135**	23.5	4.5
rainbow, grilled, 100g	–	n/a	**135**	21.5	5.4
Tuna:					
fresh, grilled, 100g	0.4	–	**170**	24.3	7.9
canned in brine, 100g	–	n/a	**99**	23.5	0.6
canned in oil, 100g	–	n/a	**189**	27.1	9

Fruit

Almost all fruits (except avocados) are low in calories, high in vitamins and fibre, and very convenient. Fruit is also high in antioxidants, which have been found to play a part in protecting the body from cancer. Wherever possible, eat fruit with the skin because of the fibre it contains.

must know

Avoid syrup

Be adventurous and try some more exotic fruits, but buy them fresh rather than tinned. Fresh is best, but if you buy tinned fruit, then never buy any in syrup – it can almost double the calorie count.

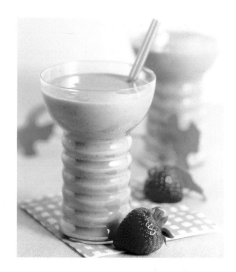

Food type	Carb (g)	Fibre (g)	Cal (kcal)	Pro (g)	Fat (g)
Apple, 1 medium	16.8	n/a	**68**	0.6	0.1
Apricots: 1 fresh	3.7	n/a	**16**	0.5	0.1
Avocado, half medium	1.6	n/a	**160**	1.6	16.4
Banana, 1 medium	23.2	n/a	**95**	1.2	0.3
Blackberries, fresh, 75g	3.8	n/a	**19**	0.7	0.2

Food type	Carb (g)	Fibre (g)	Cal (kcal)	Pro (g)	Fat (g)
Blackcurrants, fresh, 75g	5	n/a	**21**	0.7	Tr
Blueberries, fresh, 75g	7.6	1.6	**32**	0.4	0.2
Cherries, half cup fresh (90g)	10.4	0.8	**43**	0.8	0.09
Clementines, 1 medium	6.6	0.9	**28**	0.7	0.1
Figs, 1 fresh	9.6	1.7	**37**	0.4	0.2
Grapefruit, half, fresh	7.7	n/a	**34**	0.9	0.1
Grapes, black/white, seedless,					
fresh, 75g	11.6	n/a	**45**	0.3	0.1
Guavas, fresh, 60g	3	n/a	**16**	0.5	0.3
Kiwi fruit, peeled, each	10.6	n/a	**49**	1.1	0.5
Lemon, whole	3.2	n/a	**19**	1	0.3
Mangoes, 1 medium	16	n/a	**66**	0.8	0.2
Melon, fresh, medium slice:					
cantaloupe	4.9	n/a	**22**	0.7	0.1
galia	6.3	n/a	**27**	0.6	0.1
honeydew	7.5	n/a	**32**	0.7	0.1
watermelon	8	n/a	**35**	0.6	0.3
Nectarines, 1 medium	13.5	n/a	**60**	2.1	0.1
Oranges, 1 medium	12.9	n/a	**56**	1.7	0.2
Papaya, half, fresh	10	n/a	**41**	0.6	0.1
Peach, 1 medium	11.5	n/a	**50**	1.5	0.2
Pear, 1 medium	15	n/a	**60**	0.5	0.2
Pineapple, fresh, 60g	6.1	n/a	**25**	0.2	0.1
Plum, 1 medium	8.8	n/a	**36**	0.6	0.1
Raspberries, fresh, 60g	2.8	n/a	**15**	0.8	0.2
Rhubarb, fresh, raw, 60g	0.5	n/a	**4**	0.5	0.1
Satsumas, 1 medium	12.8	n/a	**54**	1.4	0.2
Strawberries, 70g	4.2	n/a	**19**	0.6	0.1
Tangerines, fresh, 1	8	n/a	**35**	0.9	0.1

Meat and poultry

The fat content of meat pushes up the calories, so always remove any visible fat and the skin of poultry. This doesn't just help your calorie count, but also reduces your overall intake of saturated fat. Watch deli meats, such as pastrami, as they are often very high-calorie; sausages are another danger area, with an average portion of two grilled beef sausages coming in at over 300 calories.

must know

Processed meats

Processed meats often contain a lot of salt as well as fat, and some have high levels of preservatives, so think about alternatives.

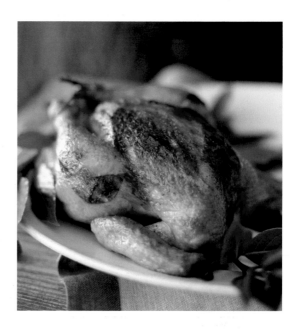

Food type	Carb (g)	Fibre (g)	Cal (kcal)	Pro (g)	Fat (g)
Bacon, 2 rashers, back (75g):					
dry fried	–	n/a	**222**	18.2	16.5
grilled	–	n/a	**216**	17.4	16.2
Beef, 100g:					
rump steak, lean, grilled	–	–	**177**	31	5.9
rump steak, lean, fried	–	–	**183**	30.9	6.6
topside, lean & fat, roasted	–	n/a	**244**	32.8	12.5
Chicken, 100g:					
breast, grilled	–	n/a	**148**	32	2.2
breast, stir fried	–	–	**161**	29.7	4.6
light & dark meat, *roasted*	–	–	**177**	27.3	7.5
light meat, roasted	–	–	**153**	30.2	3.6
cold roast chicken, breast meat, 50g	0.1	–	**76**	13.5	2.4
Ham, 50g:					
honey-roast	1.5	–	**70**	11	2.2
on the bone	0.4	0.4	**68**	10.5	3
Parma	0.1	–	**120**	12.5	7.5
Lamb, 100g:					
loin chops, lean & fat, grilled	–	–	**305**	26.5	22.1
leg, lean & fat, roasted	–	–	**240**	28.1	14.2
Pork, 100g:					
loin chops, lean, *grilled*	–	–	**184**	31.6	6.4
leg, *lean only, roasted*	–	–	**182**	33	5.5
Turkey, 100g:					
breast fillet, *grilled*	–	–	**155**	35	1.7
dark meat, roasted	–	–	**177**	29.4	6.6

Nuts, seeds and dried fruit

Measuring is essential with nuts, as they are very high in calories. Dried fruit is deceptive: though sultanas, for example, are a good addition to breakfast cereal, they can also add a lot of calories unless you are careful. Be sure you're not adding too many.

must know

Fats in nuts

The fats in nuts are generally mostly 'good' fats – mono- or polyunsaturated ones. Brazil nuts, macadamias and cashews do have significant amounts of saturated fat, and should be eaten in moderation.

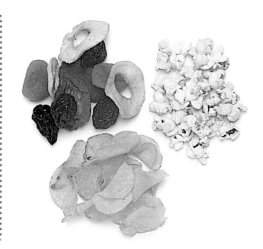

Food type	Carb (g)	Fibre (g)	Cal (kcal)	Pro (g)	Fat (g)
Almonds:					
weighed with shells, 50g	1.3	1.4	**115**	3.9	10
Apple rings, 25g	15	2.4	**60**	0.5	0.1
Apricots, 25g	9.1	n/a	**40**	1	0.2

Food type	Carb (g)	Fibre (g)	Cal (kcal)	Pro (g)	Fat (g)
Banana chips, 25g	16.2	2	**133**	0.4	7.4
Brazils:					
weighed with shells, 50g	0.7	1.9	**157**	3.3	15.7
Cashews:					
kernel only, 25g	4.5	0.8	**144**	4.5	12
Currants, 25g	17	n/a	**67**	0.6	0.1
Dates, flesh & skin, 25g	17	n/a	**68**	0.8	0.1
Figs, dried, 25g	13.2	n/a	**57**	0.9	0.4
Hazelnuts:					
weighed with shell, 50g	1.2	1.3	**124**	2.7	12.1
kernel only, 25g	1.5	1.5	**167**	4.3	16
Macadamia nuts, salted, 50g	2.4	n/a	**374**	4	38.8
Olives, 15g black	3.4	1.7	**32**	0.2	1.0
Peanuts:					
plain, weighed with shells, 50g	4.3	2.2	**195**	8.9	15.9
plain, kernel only, 25g	3.1	–	**141**	6.5	11.5
dry roasted, 50g	5.2	n/a	**295**	12.9	24.9
roasted & salted, 50g	3.6	n/a	**301**	12.4	26.5
Pine nuts, kernel only, 25g	1	n/a	**172**	3.5	17.2
Pineapple, diced, 25g	21	0.9	**87**	–	Tr
Pistachios, weighed with shells, 50g	2.3	1.7	**83**	2.5	7.7
Pumpkin seeds, 25g	3.8	1.3	**142**	6.1	11.4
Raisins, seedless, 25g	17.3	0.5	**68**	0.5	0.1
Sultanas, 25g	17.4	0.5	**69**	0.7	0.1
Sunflower seeds, 25g	4.7	1.5	**145**	55	11.9
Walnuts:					
weighed with shell, 50g	0.7	0.8	**148**	3.2	14.7
halves, 25g	0.8	0.9	**172**	3.7	17.1

Oils and fats

Though oils and fats are almost all similar in calorie value, they are not all equally good – or bad – for you; check out pages 74-7 for more information. It is essential to measure and weigh here, as a tiny error can make a big difference.

must know

Coconut and palm

Coconut oil is high in saturated fat and should be avoided, and watch out for palm oil in ingredient lists – that's also high.

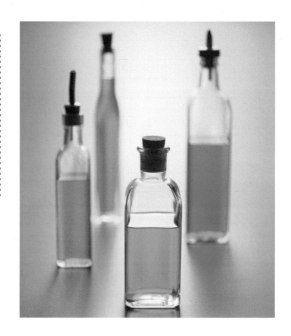

Food type	Carb (g)	Fibre (g)	Cal (kcal)	Pro (g)	Fat (g)
Butter:					
salted and unsalted, 15g	–	n/a	**111**	–	12.2
spreadable, 15g	Tr	–	**112**	0.1	12.4
Coconut oil, 1 tbsp	–	n/a	**135**	Tr	15
Ghee, 15g	Tr	n/a	**135**	Tr	15
Lard, 1 tbsp	–	n/a	**134**	Tr	14.9
Olive oil, 1 tbsp	–	n/a	**135**	Tr	15
Palm oil, 1 tbsp	–	n/a	**135**	Tr	15
Peanut oil, 1 tbsp	–	n/a	**135**	Tr	15
Rapeseed oil, 1 tbsp	–	n/a	**135**	Tr	15
Safflower oil, 1 tbsp	–	n/a	**135**	Tr	15
Sesame oil, 1 tbsp	–	n/a	**138**	–	15.3
Soya oil, 1 tbsp	–	n/a	**135**	Tr	15
Sunflower oil, 1 tbsp	–	–	**124**	–	13.8
Vegetable oil, 1 tbsp	–	–	**135**	Tr	15

Pasta, rice and noodles

There's no need to ban these from your diet so long as you watch portion sizes and measure carefully, at least in the early days. Avoid fried rice and noodles, and steer clear of most bottled pasta sauces. Check out wholemeal pasta and brown rice, which contribute more fibre; they have a gentler effect on your blood sugar.

must know

Wholemeal

Some recipes, particularly those with strong, tasty sauces, specify using wholemeal pasta. If you find one brand heavy, try another; they're not all the same.

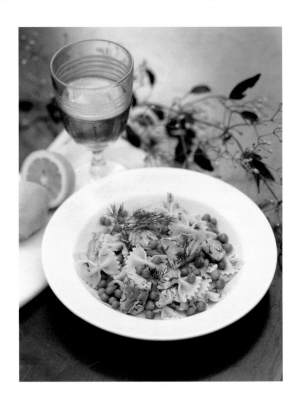

Food type	Carb (g)	Fibre (g)	Cal (kcal)	Pro (g)	Fat (g)
Pasta					
Dried pasta shapes, cooked weight 100g:					
standard	18.1	n/a	**89**	3.1	0.4
verdi	18.3	n/a	**93**	3.2	0.4
Fresh egg pasta, 100g:					
spaghetti	24	1	**129**	5	1.4
tagliatelle	24	1	**129**	5	1
Lasagne sheets, cooked weight 100g	18.1	n/a	**89**	3.1	0.4
Spaghetti, cooked weight 100g:					
dried, egg	22.2	n/a	**104**	3.6	0.7
wholemeal	23.2	n/a	**113**	4.7	0.9
Rice					
Arborio rice, 75g	23.3	0.3	**105**	2.2	0.3
Basmati rice, 75g	22.4	n/a	**113**	2	1.7
Brown rice, 75g	24	0.6	**106**	2	0.6
Egg fried rice, 75g	19.3	0.3	**156**	3.2	8
Pilau rice, 75g	23	0.5	**106**	2.7	0.4
Risotto rice, 75g	23.3	0.3	**105**	2.2	0.3
Short grain rice, 75g	26	0.7	**108**	2	0.3
White rice, plain, 75g	23.2	0.1	**104**	2	1
Wholegrain rice, 75g	21.2	0.6	**102**	2.7	0.7
Noodles					
Egg noodles, 75g	9.8	0.5	**47**	2	0.4
Thai rice noodles, 75g	26	0.7	**108**	2	0.3
Thread noodles, 75g	7.4	–	**51**	1.8	1.5

Sugar and chocolate

Try to reduce your intake of sugar, and experiment with fructose – fruit sugar, now easily available. It has the same calorie count as sugar but you need much less, only about 65g where you would use 100g of sugar. Dark chocolate can be a delicious treat, but make sure you can stop at a reasonable amount, and don't forget to add the calories to your daily total.

must know

Hidden sugar

There can be a lot of sugar in processed food and ready meals, sometimes in the most surprising places. Check ingredient labels carefully and avoid anything high in sugar.

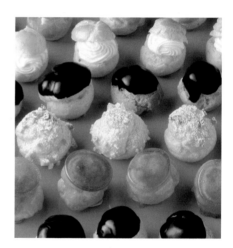

Food type	Carb (g)	Fibre (g)	Cal (kcal)	Pro (g)	Fat (g)
Amber sugar crystals, 1 tsp	5	–	20	Tr	–
Chocolate, 25g:					
milk	14.2	n/a	130	1.9	7.7
plain	15.9	n/a	128	1.3	7
white	14.6	n/a	132	2	7.7
Date syrup, 1 tsp	3.7	Tr	15	0.1	–
Fructose, 1 tsp	5	–	20	–	–
Golden syrup, 1 tsp	4	–	15	–	–
Honey, 1 tsp:					
clear	3.7	n/a	15	–	Tr
set	3.5	–	14	–	–
Icing sugar, 1 tsp	5	–	20	–	–
Jaggery	4.8	n/a	18	–	–
Maple syrup, 1 tsp	4.2	Tr	17	Tr	–
Molasses, 1 tsp	4	–	16	–	–
Sugar:					
caster, 1 tsp	5	–	20	–	–
cube, white, each	5	–	20	–	–
dark brown, soft, 1 tsp	4.8	–	19	–	–
demerara, cane, 1 tsp	5	Tr	20	Tr	–
granulated, 1 tsp	5	–	20	–	–
light brown, soft, 1 tsp	4.7	–	19	–	–
preserving, 1 tsp	5	–	20	–	–
Treacle, black, 1 tsp	3.3	n/a	13	0.1	–

Vegetables

Most vegetables won't have an alarming effect on your diet, provided they're not drowning in butter or oil, fried or served in creamy sauces. Watch out for potatoes and other starchy vegetables like cassava, which need careful weighing. Sweetcorn and peas can also be surprisingly high-cal, so be a bit cautious with them.

must know

Cooking

Overcooking destroys many nutrients in vegetables, so cook them for the minimum amount of time and in as little liquid as possible.

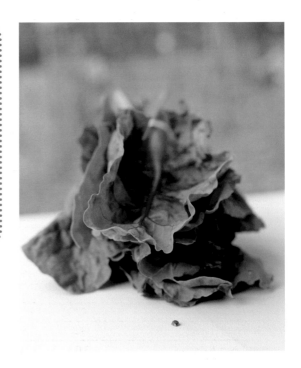

Food type	Carb (g)	Fibre (g)	Cal (kcal)	Pro (g)	Fat (g)
Artichokes, 1 globe	2.7	–	**18**	2.8	0.2
Asparagus, 6 spears, boiled	1.1	n/a	**21**	2.7	0.6
Aubergine, half medium, fried	1.4	n/a	**151**	0.6	16
Beans, broad, boiled, 75g	8.8	n/a	**61**	5.9	0.5
Beans, French, 100g boiled	4.7	n/a	**25**	1.7	0.1
Beans, runner, 50g, trimmed, boiled	1.2	n/a	**9**	0.6	0.3
Beetroot, 90g:					
trimmed, peeled	7	n/a	**32**	1.5	0.1
pickled	23.4	n/a	**98**	0.9	0.1
Broccoli, florets, boiled, 60g	0.7	n/a	**14**	1.9	0.5
Brussels sprouts, 6 trimmed, boiled	4.9	n/a	**49**	4.1	0.6
Cabbage (Savoy, Summer), 75g:					
trimmed	3.1	n/a	**20**	1.3	0.3
Spring greens, raw	2.3	n/a	**25**	2.3	0.8
white	3.7	1.6	**20**	1.0	0.2
Carrot:					
1 medium, raw	7.9	n/a	**35**	0.6	0.3
1 medium, raw (young)	6.8	n/a	**34**	0.8	0.6
grated, 40g	3.2	1	**15**	0.2	0.1
boiled (young), 80g	3.5	n/a	**18**	0.5	0.3
Cassava, 100g:					
baked	40.1	1.7	**155**	0.7	0.2
boiled	33.5	1.4	**130**	0.5	0.2
Cauliflower, 100g, raw	3.0	n/a	**34**	3.6	0.9
Celeriac, 100g, flesh only, boiled	1.9	3.2	**15**	0.9	0.5
Celery, 100g, stem only, raw	0.9	n/a	**7**	0.5	0.2
Corn-on-the-cob, boiled, 1 medium	13.3	n/a	**76**	2.9	1.6
Courgettes (zucchini), raw 50g	0.9	n/a	**9**	0.9	0.2
Cucumber, trimmed, 75g	1.1	n/a	**8**	0.5	0.2

Food type	Carb (g)	Fibre (g)	Cal (kcal)	Pro (g)	Fat (g)
Fennel, Florence, boiled, 75g	1.1	n/a	**8**	0.7	0.2
Garlic, half tsp purée or					
1 clove, crushed	1.8	0.9	**60**	0.4	5.7
Ginger root, half tsp, grated	1	0.1	-	-	-
Kale, curly, boiled, 40g	0.4	n/a	**10**	1	0.4
Leeks, *boiled*, 100g	2.6	n/a	**21**	1.2	0.7
Lettuce, 1 cup (30g):					
green	0.5	n/a	**4**	0.2	0.2
iceberg	0.6	n/a	**4**	0.2	0.1
mixed leaf	0.8	0.8	**5**	0.3	0.03
Mediterranean salad leaves	0.9	0.5	**6**	0.3	0.1
spinach, rocket & watercress	0.4	0.4	**7.5**	0.9	0.3
Mange-tout, 50g:					
raw	2.1	n/a	**16**	1.8	0.1
Mushrooms, common, 40g:					
raw	0.2	n/a	**5**	0.7	0.2
Mushrooms, oyster, 30g	-	0.1	**2**	0.5	0.1
Okra (gumbo, ladies' fingers):					
raw, 25g	2	-	**10**	0.5	-
Onions, raw, flesh only, 30g	2.4	n/a	**11**	0.4	0.1
Parsnips, trimmed, peeled,					
boiled, 80g	10.3	n/a	**53**	1.3	1.0
Peas:					
fresh, raw, 75g	8.5	n/a	**62**	5.1	1.1
Peppers:					
green, raw, 40g	1.0	n/a	**6**	0.3	0.1
red, raw, 40g	2.6	n/a	**13**	0.4	0.2
yellow, raw, 40g	2.1	0.7	**10**	0.5	0.1
chilli, 15g	0.1	n/a	**3**	0.4	0.1

Food type	Carb (g)	Fibre (g)	Cal (kcal)	Pro (g)	Fat (g)
Potatoes, new, 100g:					
boiled, peeled	17.8	n/a	75	1.5	0.3
boiled in skins	15.4	n/a	66	1.4	0.3
Potatoes, old, 180g (1 medium):					
baked, flesh & skin	57	n/a	244	7	0.4
baked, flesh only	32.4	n/a	138	4.0	0.2
boiled, peeled	30.6	n/a	130	3.2	0.2
Pumpkin, flesh only, boiled, 75g	1.7	n/a	10	0.5	0.2
Raddicchio, 30g	0.5	0.5	4	0.4	0.1
Radish, red, 6	1.1	n/a	7	0.4	0.1
Radish, white/mooli, 20g	0.6	–	3	0.2	–
Salsify, flesh only, boiled, 50g	4.3	1.8	12	0.6	0.2
Shallots, 30g	1.0	n/a	6	0.5	0.1
Spinach:					
raw, one cup, 30g	0.5	n/a	8	0.8	0.2
Spring onions, bulbs & tops, 30g	0.9	n/a	7	0.6	0.2
Squash:					
flesh only, 50g	1.1	n/a	6	0.3	0.1
Swede, flesh only, boiled, 90g	2.1	n/a	10	0.3	0.1
Sweet potato, boiled, 90g	18.5	n/a	76	1.0	0.3
Sweetcorn, kernels, 80g	21.3	n/a	98	2.3	1.0
Tomatoes:					
1 medium	4.7	0.6	29	1.1	0.6
canned, whole, 100g	3	n/a	16	1	0.1
cherry, 6	5.3	1.7	31	1.2	0.5
sundried, 30g	3.3	2	63	1.3	4.9
Turnip, flesh only, boiled, 60g	1.2	n/a	7	0.4	0.1
Water chestnuts, canned, 40g	1.9	1	11	0.7	0.1
Yam, flesh only, boiled, 90g	29.7	n/a	120	1.5	0.3

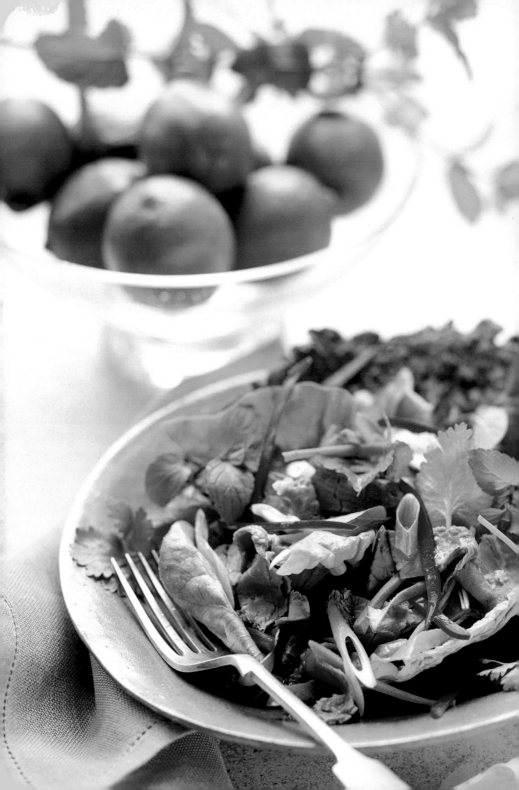

Appendices

Further reading

General nutrition

Bodyfoods for Busy People, Jane Clarke, 2004

Collins Gem Calorie Counter, 2004

Collins Gem What Diet?, 2005

Collins Gem GI Guide, 2005

Eat, Drink and Be Healthy, Walter Willett, 2001

Eat Well, Live Well series, recipe books, various authors

Fat is a Feminist Issue, Susie Orbach, 1998

Food Pharmacy, Jean Carper, 2000

A Good Life, Leo Hickman, 2005

L is for Label: How to Read Between the Lines on Food Packaging, Amanda Ursell, 2004

Low-Calorie Dieting for Dummies, Susan McQuillan, 2005

Nutrition for Dummies, Nigel Denby, Sue Baic and Carol Ann Rinzler, 2005

Nutrition for Life, Ian W. Campbell, 2005

Patrick Holford's New Optimum Nutrition Bible, Patrick Holford, 2004

Think Well to be Well, Azmina Govindji, 2002

Vitamins and Minerals Handbook, Amanda Ursell, et al, 2001

The Weight-Loss Bible, Joanna Hall, 2005

GI/GL diets

The GI Diet, by Rick Gallop, 2004

The Low GI Diet, by Jennie Brand-Miller & Kaye Foster-Powell with Joanna McMillan-Price, 2004

Collins NTK GI + GL Diet, 2006

Collins Gem GL, 2006

Recipe books

Classic 1000 Calorie-counted Recipes, Carolyn Humphries, 1998

Healthy Eating for Diabetics, Antony Worrall Thompson & Azmina Govindji, 2003

Healthy Mediterranean Cooking, Rena Salaman, 1999

The High-Energy Cookbook, by Rachael Anne Hill, 2004

Jane Clarke's Bodyfoods Cookbook: Recipes for Life, Jane Clarke, 2001

Reader's Digest Low Calorie Cookbook, 2003

Exercise

Collins Gem Pilates, 2003

Collins Gem Yoga, 2003

Fitness for Life, Matt Roberts, 2002

The Exercise Bible, Joanna Hall, 2003

The Pilates Directory, Alan Herdman, 2004

Workouts for Dummies, Tamilee Webb, 1998

Useful addresses

British Dietetic Association
5th Floor, Charles House
148-9 Great Charles Street
Queensway
Birmingham B3 3HT
www.bda.uk.com

British Heart Foundation
14 Fitzhardinge Street
London W1H 6DH
020 7935 0185

British Nutrition Foundation
High Holborn House
52-54 High Holborn
London WC1V 6RQ
020 7404 6504

Coronary Prevention Group
2 Taviton Street
London WC1
020 7927 2125
www.healthnet.org

Diabetes UK
10 Parkway
London NW1 7AA
Careline 0845 1202960
or 020 7424 1000 and ask to
be transferred to the Careline

Eating Disorders Association,
1 Prince of Wales Rd,
Norwich, NR1 1DW,
www.edauk.com
Tel: 0845 634 1414 (adult
helpline); 0845 634 7650
(youth helpline)

Institute for Optimum Nutrition
Blades Court, Deodar Road
London SW15 2NU
020 8877 9993
No nutrition advice given but
they will recommend a
nutritionist

The Vegetarian Society
Parkdale,
Dunham Rd,
Altrincham,
Cheshire, WA14 4QG
www.vegsoc.org

Women's Health Concern
PO Box 2126
Marlow
Bucks SL7 2PU
Tel. 0845 1232319 to speak to
a nurse
or 01628 488065 for other
information
www.womens-health-concern.org

Picture credits

Photos copyright © Getty Images:

Victor Budknik/Cole Group pp. 36, 134; Patricia Brabant/Cole Group pp. 61, 180; Michael Lamotte/Cole Group p. 77; D. Fischer & P. Lyons/Cole Group p. 101; Chris Shorten/Cole Group p. 108; Keith Ovregaard/Cole Group pp. 111, 133; Kevin Sanchez/Cole Group p. 139 (top); Jackson Vereen/Cole Group pp. 143, 145; Chris Shorten/Cole Group p. 144; Dennis Gray/Cole Group pp. 152, 168

Photos copyright © Photodisc:

Ryan McVay pp. 13, 22, 30, 38, 50, 51, 54, 99; Nancy R. Cohen pp. 15, 46, 65, 136; Jules Frazier pp. 16, 41, 56 (both); Duncan Smith pp. 26, 31, 90, 91, 98, 176; David Buffington pp. 34, 52; Nick Rower pp. 45; Karl Weatherly pp. 49; Mitch Hrdlicka pp. 53, 75, 80, 149, 162, 164

Photos copyright © Jupiter Images:

Brian Hagiwara & Jonelle Weaver/Brand X: pp. 2, 6, 8, 10, 11, 20, 32, 58, 66, 67, 69, 70, 73, 83, 84, 86, 89, 93, 105, 106, 110, 112, 114, 117, 119, 120, 121, 122, 124, 126, 129, 137, 153, 156, 158, 160, 166, 170, 172, 174, 178, 182, 186

Photo by Christina Jansen, copyright © Grapevine Publishing Services:

p. 74, 174

Graphics by Judith Ash, copyright © Grapevine Publishing Services:

Pp. 28, 64

Index

A

alcohol 11, 82-4, 94, 97, 166-7
Alexander Technique 55
antioxidants 68, 82, 153, 154, 170
arthritis 43
avocado 111, 170

B

balanced diet 62-3
bananas 66-7
beans 69, 127, 160
Bean salad 129
beef 71
steak 65, 121
Hot beef stir-fry 134
beer 84
bingeing 104-5
blood pressure 31, 34, 56, 75, 78
blood-sugar levels 12-13, 21, 64, 71, 77, 94, 178
Body Mass Index (BMI) 26, 28-31, 36
boredom 10, 106
boxercise 51
bread 64, 99, 158-9
Lebanese bread salad 130
breakfast 116
cereals 162-3
build 24-5

C

caffeine 82
calcium 72
cancer 35, 43, 66, 170
carbohydrates 63-8
cardiovascular disease 34, 168

carrots
Carrot and ginger soup 128
cheese 93, 102, 111
Grilled goat's cheese on mushrooms 132
Roquefort and pear salad 131
chicken 71, 120
Chicken with mushrooms and tomatoes 147
Oriental chicken with lemon, ginger, garlic and soy 148
chickpeas 161
Spicy chickpea, spinach and aubergine casserole 138
children 36-7
chocolate 12, 98, 122, 123, 180-1
cholesterol 77
coffee 81, 82, 166
condiments 76
cooking 99-103, 182
courgettes 140
crash diets 14
cream 67, 72, 111, 167
fake 151
cycling 48
dairy products 72, 74, 164-5
desserts 111, 121-3
Apple and orange fool 151
Baked oranges with cinnamon and Cointreau 155

Baked peaches with amaretti biscuits 152
Plum compôte 154
Refreshing mango and citrus salad 153

D

diabetes 12, 34, 43, 46, 189
diet addiction 34
digestion 10-11, 17
dressings 111, 118
dried fruit 96, 174-5
drinks 81-4, 97, 166-7

E

eating disorders 33, 108, 189
eating out 103, 110-111
eggs 63, 71, 164-5
Tunisian eggs 136
European Protective Investigation of Cancer (EPIC) 68
exercise 17-18, 40-48, 188
aerobic 32, 48-9
anaerobic/resistance 50-1
at work 54-5
at home 56
benefits of 56-7

F

farmers' markets 61
fats 74-7
hydrogenated/trans 76
in nuts 174
saturated 76-7
unsaturated 74-5
fibre 13, 62, 64, 68
fish and seafood 72, 168-9

Baked fish (cod) and chips with tomato salsa 144
canned 168
Keralan prawn curry 141
oily 73, 75
Roast salmon with courgettes 140
Smoked haddock fishcakes 142
Tuna and chive pâté 146
fizzy drinks 81, 166
food diary 88-90
food labels 76, 78, 80, 98
frame size 24-7
fructose 81, 180
fruit 65-7, 122-3, 170-1
Apple and orange fool 151
Baked oranges with cinnamon and Cointreau 155
Baked peaches with amaretti biscuits 152
dried 96, 174-5
juices 164-5
Pear and Roquefort salad 131
Plum compôte 154
purées 102
Refreshing mango and citrus salad 153

G

gardening 45, 56
glucose 11-12, 40, 64
glycaemic index (GI) 80
GI diets 63-4, 188
glycaemic load (GL) 63, 80, 188

Appendices

H

heart disease 12, 43, 46, 77, 189
height/weight chart 27

I

insulin 12-13, 77, 85
insulin resistance syndrome 12

J

junk food 37, 60

L

leeks
    Leek, potato and saffron soup 129
lentils 67, 160-1
    Lentil, onion and coriander soup 126
lunch 118-19

M

main meals 119-121
maintaining weight 112-13
malnutrition 19, 20
mangoes 153
measuring spoons 100
meat and poultry 71, 172-3
    processed meats 172
meringue 111, 121
metabolism 16-17
milk 72, 92
minerals 78-9
motivation 33-5
muscle 13, 14, 52
    building 18, 40, 43, 50
mushrooms 132
    dried 147

N

non-stick pans 100
noodles 178-9
nutrition 74, 188
nuts 70, 174-5

O

oats 65
oatcakes 118, 123, 159
oil 75-6, 101, 176-7
    oil spray 132
olives 104
omega-3 fats 75, 168
osteoporosis 43

P

parties 109
pasta 63, 102, 178-9
    Tomato and rocket pasta 135
pastry 111
pedometers 44, 46
Pilates 51, 55
plums 154
pork 71
    Sautéed pork fillet with herbs and white wine 150
posture 55
potatoes 66, 71, 129, 182, 185
prawns 121
    Keralan prawn curry 141
processed food 60, 61, 76, 100, 172, 180
protein 68-74
    deficiency 69-70
pulses 67-8, 160-1

Q

quinoa 65, 69

R

raspberries 96
record-keeping 94-7
resting metabolic rate (RMR) 13-18
rice 63, 65, 120, 178-9
    Valpolicella risotto 137

S

salads 111, 118
    Bean salad 129
    Grilled goat's cheese on mushrooms 132
    Lebanese bread salad 130
    Pear and Roquefort salad 131
    Salade Niçoise 118
    Warm lentil, bacon and spinach salad 133
salt 76, 78-80
sandwiches 67, 119, 148, 158
sardines 64
sausages 172
seeds 75, 174-5
shopping 97-9
snacks 47, 67, 77, 97, 123
soups 101
    Carrot and ginger soup 128
    Leek, potato and saffron soup 129
    Lentil, onion and coriander soup 126
    Tomato and red pepper soup 127
soya products 69
spinach 103, 133, 138
spirits 83, 84, 97, 167
sports bras 52
sports drinks 40
stroke 34, 65, 77, 78
sugar 80-1, 98, 180-1
sweeteners 81
swimming 48

T

tea 81, 82, 166
thyroid, underactive 17, 21

TV time 36, 37, 44, 49

V

vegetables 65-7, 70, 182-3
vegetarians 69, 189
vitamins 78-9

W

waist to hip ratio 30
waist size 31
walking 45-8
    using pedometer 44, 46
water 52, 68, 81
weighing yourself 11, 28, 90-1
whole grains 63, 64, 65, 68
wine 18, 21, 84, 123

Y

yoga 51
yo-yo dieting 16, 19